Concentrated
Fat–Burners

Concentrated Fat–Burners

William H. Lee, R.Ph., Ph.D.

Instant Improvement, Inc.

Instant Improvement, Inc.
1160 Park Avenue
New York, New York 10128

Manufactured in the United States of America

Library of Congress Cataloging–in–Publication Data

Lee, William H.
    Concentrated fat–burners

    Bibliography: p.
    Includes index.
    1. Reducing.   2. Dietary supplements.   3. Amino
acids—Therapeutic use.   4. Vitamins—Therapeutic use.
I. Title.
RM222.2.L417   1988   616.3'98061   87–34819
ISBN 0–941683–01–X

IMPORTANT NOTICE

This book contains material for informational and educational purposes only. It seeks to make people aware of their health needs.

If any person makes a decision to use any data found in this book, the decision rests completely with that person and his or her own doctor.

This book is not a substitute for personal medical supervision by a qualified health professional. People with health problems should consult with their physicians.

Any action taken by any reader concerning therapies or individual substances rests solely with the reader and his or her doctor.

*Dedicated to the two people who have
no need for this book:
Lynn and Fredda*

*With a special thanks to Mel Rich
for all of the research material*

A Public Note of Thanks

To the many physicians, dieticians, nutritionists, researchers, and other health professionals whose knowledge and insights went toward the preparation of this book—in journals such as these:

American Journal of Clinical Nutrition

American Journal of Medicine, The

American Journal of Physiology

Annual Review of Nutrition

Archives of Biochemical Biophysics

Biochemical Pharmacology

Biological Trace Element Research

European Journal of Applied Physiology

Gastroenterology

International Clinical Nutrition Review

Journal of the American Dietetic Association

Journal of the American Medical Association

Journal of Clinical Psychiatry

Journal of the International Academy of Nutritional Consultants, The

Journal of Nutrition

Journal of Nutrition and Metabolism

Journal of Nutritional Science

Journal of Pharmacology and Experimental Therapy

Lancet, The

Life Sciences

Medical Tribune

Metabolism

Nutrition Review

Review of Physiological Chemistry

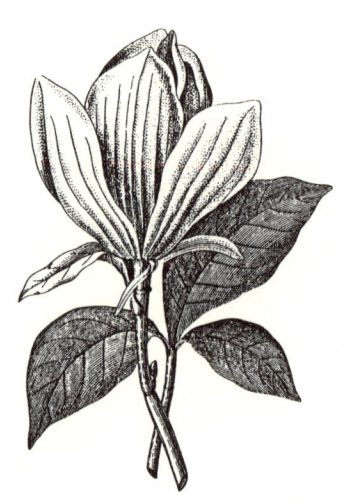

Table of Contents

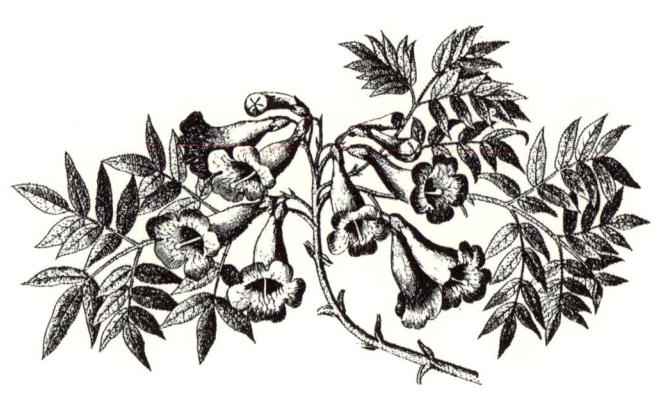

Diet Panic and Stress Panic

Why is it that many people can eat everything they want and still look like models strolling down a runway?

How much does heredity have to do with your weight?

Blame it on a slow metabolism? "It's my thyroid gland that keeps me fat!"

The truth is, many factors get together in your body to determine whether you'll be fat or skinny. *And, you can't control your weight unless you learn all of the facts, understand the whole story—and then change all of the factors under your control.*

There are products on the market that can help you. You won't need a doctor's prescription to buy them. They're available in every health food store and drugstore. However, you do have to know your own body in order to choose the product that will benefit you the most.

Here's a quick rundown on fat–facts and theories to help you begin to understand your own body.

Why Do We Get Fat?

For an answer to this question we have to go back fifteen thousand years or more. Humans were just beginning to evolve into the "modern" men and women we see walking the streets today. Life was hard, and most waking hours were spent in finding enough food to sustain life. The rest of the hours were spent in finding safe shelter. Man did not know how to store food during the warm months, and, even if he did, storage facilities were limited to the back of a cave. The idea of drying grains and seeds so they would last over the winter months had not yet occurred to ancient tribes, and the fact that cold months and warm months happened with regularity was not yet fully understood.

In that beginning culture the only guarantee of getting through the winter was to acquire a heavy layer of body fat. Women, because they had to bear the young to keep the race from dying out, were usually fatter than the men.

But Why Are There Fat Women and Skinny Women?

Everyone is born with a certain number of fat cells. Genetics play the biggest part in how many fat cells you acquire at birth. If your ancestors were among the fattest in the cave, they survived the toughest winters and passed their genes on to succeeding generations, ending up with you.

Why did the skinny women survive that tough winter? Maybe they attracted the best hunter in the cave, or were able to sit nearest the fire, or maybe they lived in a more temperate zone.

Whichever, everyone is born with a designated number of fat cells according to an individual genetic plan.

How Can I Get Rid of My Fat Cells?

The answer is—you can't. Not only are your fat cells permanent, but you can add to them. If you are excessively heavy, your body will manufacture *new* fat cells. Like the ones you were born with, the new fat cells will never disappear. And, fat cells are designed to store fat.

Does That Mean "Once Fat—Always Fat"?

No way!

Fat cells can be made to shrink. Flatten out. Be almost invisible. That's the fatty's goal, and it's not impossible once you understand how you can influence your own biological tendencies.

Maybe It's My Metabolism?

If you want to blame your obesity on your metabolism, you'll never lose weight. You're using a crutch to make yourself feel better.

You may have a slow metabolism, but it isn't your metabolism that's making you fat. You have a slow metabolism because you're fat! Part of the problem is that you went on a very restricted–calorie diet.

Should I Blame My Diet?

Yes, or rather what your diet stimulated in your body. For that explanation we have once again to go back fifteen thousand years.

Enter Diet Panic

Many of the problems we face in this day and age can be traced back to the fact that the human body has changed very little since the cave days. We still eat food, need sunlight, bear young, and live in caves (we call them apartments or houses). Although physically our environment does not resemble the world of our remote ancestors, our bodies are essentially the same, and react in a similar manner to many of the same problems.

One of the problems is the safety of the race. The "old brain," the one that controls our basic needs and desires—like safety, sex, anger, all of the so-called "primitive" emotions, is alive and well and living in our bodies.

This "old brain" is very concerned about our health as individuals and about the health of our human race.

Normally, we enjoy a regulating mechanism, the "new brain," a "younger" brain, which evolved at a later period. The actual location of this regulator is in the hypothalamus. Our regulating mechanism, when it is operating as it should, helps to keep our weight on an even keel, at the level at which we feel most comfortable. It is called our "set point."

This mechanism balances caloric input against energy output. If we eat too much at one meal it helps us to eat less at the next meal, or it initiates exercise (an increase in energy output) to make up for the extra calories. When it is working well it helps to keep our weight constant—whether at normal weight or beyond it.

And then we decide to go on a diet! We cut our food intake drastically—from 3,500 calories of food to 1,200 calories of food. And Diet Panic sets in.

"Famine!"

"Begin emergency procedures!"

You have to understand that Diet Panic results from a lack of nutrients. You understand that you want to lose weight. But your body only knows that it was used to getting a load of vitamins, minerals, trace elements, protein, fat, and carbohydrates, and now that plentiful supply has been reduced by more than half.

The Diet Panic takes over metabolism and fat storage.

The regulating mechanism is instructed to start storing more fat and using less energy.

A greater proportion of the smaller amount of food you are now eating is stored away in the fat cells and less fat is burned for energy.

15

Can We Get Around Diet Panic?

Sure, by using nutritional magic and some of the substances available to help soothe its anguish.

But first, there's another problem you should be aware of. It's called Stress Panic.

Another Legacy from Our Cave Days?

Right on. And this phenomenon is also responsible for the way we lose or gain weight.

What Is This One and What Does It Do?

As humans were evolving back in those early days, a complex set of physiological reactions were built into the body to handle the effects of stress. In those prehistoric days stress usually arose from physical danger, with the threat of death at every turn. Early humans reacted to this stress with explosive *action.*

Our bodies today still respond without conscious thought. The lungs and heart rush extra oxygen to the muscles, the pupils dilate for better vision, the muscles tense up for exertion, and the bloodstream is flooded with special hormones. The liver releases glucose for energy, and fat for extra fuel is dumped from the fat cells.

This famous "flight or fight" reaction is designed to save our lives in times of stress or danger. Without this unconscious reflex action, mankind might not have been able to overcome primitive disasters.

As modern people we also are stressed, but the stress we face in our lives is seldom physical. Rather it can be a pile of unpaid bills, an audit by the IRS, an irate boss, or bumper–to–bumper traffic. Fighting or running seldom helps these problems. We usually just smile and suppress our feelings.

But fear and anxiety sill trigger the same stress reactions, as if we had come face–to–face with a saber–toothed tiger!

Heart rate and breathing still increase. Hormones are still released. Sugar and fat are still dumped into the bloodstream. And the body is still prepared for action.

That's when Stress Panic goes to work.

When no action takes place to use up all of those potential "fight or flight" substances, Diet Stress gathers all of them up and, you guessed it, stores them all away as fat!

And do you know what stresses the body most? *Dieting*!

So now you know about the two factors that work against your losing weight:

Diet Panic with its fear of famine, and Diet Stress, with its reluctance to lose any nourishment. These two factors keep most diets from working.

All of the popular diets call for drastic reductions in the amount of food you eat. And they suggest a lot of exercise. So you eat less and sweat a lot—and drop a pound or two. Then Diet Panic and Diet Stress wake up and you're back where you started when you step on the scale—or maybe you're even a pound or two heavier!

If eating less and sweating are the only answers to the diet problem, why are there so many hungry fat people bathed in perspiration?

This is not a diet book in the true sense of the word. In this book there will be no endless lists of foods to avoid, or foods you must eat, or calorie tables, or recipes. There will be none of that at all. Instead, what you will find in this book is how to get around the natural forces in your body that work against your losing weight.

There are many good diets presented in many good books. *Concentrated Fat–Burners* will be compatible with *any* intelligent weight–loss program and *any* good exercise program (both are necessary for weight loss).

There are nutritional aids that can come between you and Diet Panic. These aids can persuade Diet Panic to relax its dictatorial policy.

There are nutrients that can replace the ones spent by the body on ineffectual responses to stress.

There are methods to increase so–called Brown Fat at the expense of White Fat (Brown Fat burns up White Fat for energy).

Concentrated Fat–Burners presents all of the products and separate substances that are available to you. Since people are individuals, although sharing many of the same needs and problems, there is not product or substance that is superior to all of the others. What will work in one case may not in another; so, you may have to try one approach and then another to find the ideal one for you.

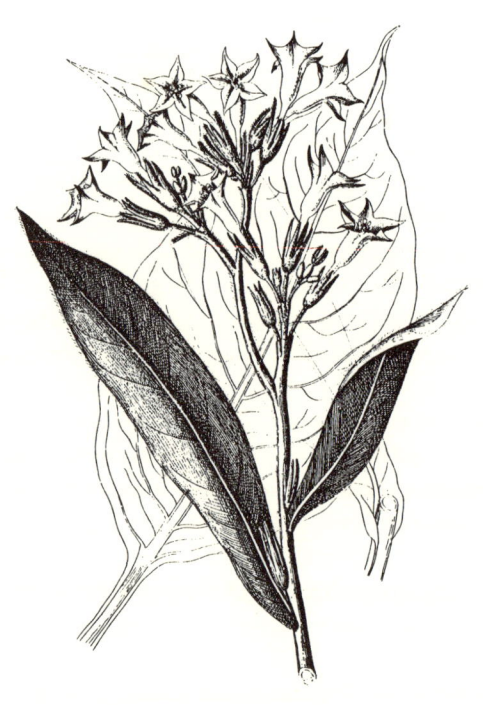

Appetite Is In Your Mind

Better Living through Brain Chemistry

Appetite, like sex, it is said, begins in the mind. This is a statement that is a little like the chicken–and–egg paradox. Do brain chemicals influence the emotions or do the emotions influence production of brain chemicals—and what's the difference?

First, examine love at first sight: strangers look at each other and are attracted. The attraction stimulates brain chemicals (neurotransmitters) and a rapturous feeling floods the body.

They kiss!

According to British researchers, the kiss is a "tasting" procedure where each person samples the other's semio–chemicals secreted by special glands in the mouth area. If they like the "taste" they go on to explore other activities until satiated.

Chemicals manufactured by the body play an important role in the affair. How often have you heard that two people have "the same chemistry"? How often has love been described as "a chemical reaction"?

Appetite also begins in the brain! The brain monitors all physical activities and requires an adequate amount of fuel to keep the body running as it should. When fuel is low (food is fuel), the brain sends out commands to eat. *These commands are in the form of neurotransmitters of brain chemicals.*

When there is a sufficient amount of high–grade fuel in the body *the brain produces another neurotransmitter, which tells the body to stop eating*!

True hunger is the result of chemicals manufactured by the brain. Normal eating is also the result of brain chemicals. Feeling full and the command to stop eating is an end product of chemistry. So—it should be possible to lose weight and control your appetite by resorting to chemical principles!

And it is.

You can manipulate the neurotransmitters in your brain, and outwit Diet Panic. You can reach your dream weight without ever resorting to agonizing diets—or dangerous drugs and prescriptions.

Nutrients are different from drugs.

A nutrient is a food substance that, in most cases, supplies either building blocks the body needs to make cells and tissue, or energy the body needs to keep its mechanism functioning.

Drugs, on the other hand, work on a particular organ or cell.

All healthy people, obese or otherwise, must have the same nutrients, whereas a drug would be recommended only if there is a particular disease or condition to be treated.

However, under special circumstances, when nutrients are taken in food or as supplements, they can give rise to important changes in the chemicals manufactured by the body.

And that principle can mean the difference between the success or failure of your weight–lose program!

In early days, before the concept that nutrition is an important factor in daily living, we assumed that what we ate had little effect on brain function, since the adult brain contained its own means to synthesize chemicals according to need. Now it appears that neurotransmitter synthesis in the brain is not as autonomous as once believed. The type of food offered to the body as fuel, and its protein content, can influence the manufacture of those brain chemicals.

Protein (from the Greek word "proteios," which literally translates to mean the most fundamental matter), carbohydrates, and fats are three life–sustaining nutrients. Living cells are manufactured from protein. The other two nutrients supply energy.

The proteins you get from meat, milk, eggs, rice, and other sources are first fragmented in the digestive tract into the amino acids. All protein is composed of chains of amino acids, from only a few to thousands, linked together in specific ways. There are as many patterns as can be imagined. As we look at bacteria, plants, animals, and humans, the same amino acids appear, but in diverse quantities and shapes. The higher we go in the evolutionary chain, the more complicated the patterns.

Nevertheless, all food protein is broken down into the individual amino acids, which are then reassembled into patterns needed by the body.

Scientists tell us that there are basically twenty–two amino acids. Eight of the twenty–two are growth and maintenance chemicals, and are absolutely essential constituents of an adequate diet. These eight cannot be manufactured by the body, but must be obtained either from food or from supplements. All of the other amino acids, called nonessential amino acids, can be made by the body cells from fats or carbohydrates combined with nitrogen.

What Does This Have To Do with Dieting and Losing Weight?

The brain uses certain amino acids as raw material in the manufacture of brain chemicals. When these amino acids are obtained from food, they are carried to the brain to pass through the blood–brain barrier into the brain area. The blood–brain barrier is a protective device that prevents unwanted substances from invading the brain area.

Since most amino acids derived from food approach the brain area in more or less equal amounts and have to use the same "ferry–molecules" to cross the barrier, there is usually not much more of one amino acid than another.

We can now load the dice in favor of natural appetite suppression

We do this in two ways:

First, by coaxing the brain to manufacture more and more of a special little chemical—one that prevents the Diet Panic that stops the body from burning fat.

And then we can go on, and convince the brain to make more of the chemical that says we have had enough to eat.

So we feel great. We feel full. And the fat is melting off our bodies like butter.

One of the problems with a low–calorie approach to dieting is feeling deprived and hungry.

You may be getting an adequate amount of nutrients (if you are also taking supplementary vitamins and minerals) but the empty feeling and Diet Panic work against you.

Nutritional manipulation of brain chemicals can change the situation and strengthen your resolve to lose weight.

The amino acids involved in this particular nutritional approach are available in supplement form at your health food store or drugstore.

Phenylalanine

This is one of the essential amino acids that can help you control your appetite without becoming depressed. It is 100 percent natural. Phenylalanine is found in many foods, particularly in meats and milk. When it reaches the brain it is turned into a neurotransmitter (a chemical that is able to transmit signals between the nerve cells and the brain).

If It Is Natural and I Can Get It from Food, Why Should I Buy It in a Supplement Form? I Could Just Eat and Get Thin!

That would be nice. If you could eat yourself thin there would be no obesity and no need for this book. The problem is the competition between all of the amino acids to get into the brain area.

Foods contain a number of amino acids. Meats and dairy products contain *all* of the essential amino acids and all of them are digested at the same time and approach the brain at the same time.

Because there is a more or less even distribution of the amino acids, there is an even effect on the production of brain chemicals.

Isn't That the Way It's Supposed to Be?

Sure it is if you want to be at the mercy of Diet Panic and Stress Panic when you desire to lose weight. However, if you want to exert control over your own weight, you have to do more than just cut down on food and increase the amount of exercise you do. You have to induce your brain to work *with* you.

And that can be done with nutritional magic!

You will not be taking chemicals or drugs that are harmful; you will be using natural substances found in food. However, you will use them in their concentrated form as tablets or capsules.

What Does Phenylalanine Do?

First, we have to put an "L" in front of the phenylalanine. That's to distinguish it from D–Phenylalanine.

Amino acids are crystal in substance, and the letter "L" stands for levorotary, meaning that when this particular amino acid is placed in solution and a beam of light is directed at it, the molecules will rotate to the left.

"D" is the abbreviation for dextrorotary, which tells us that the molecules will rotate to the right. Levo—left; dextro—right.

The "L" form is important because with almost all of the amino acids you will use, it is the "L" form that works best in the body. You'll have to read the label on the supplement bottle to make sure you are getting the right form.

O.K., Now That I Know What to Buy, What Does It Do; How Much Do I Take; and When Do I Take It?

When L–phenylalanine is able to cross the barrier into the brain in a larger than normal concentration, it is turned into noradrenaline and dopamine, two neurotransmitters. L–phenylalanine→noradrenaline (norepinephrine)→dopamine.

These brain chemicals tend to tilt the mental mood toward excitement, alertness, sexual awareness, and they also tend to help the body control appetite. L–phenylalanine invites the release of a hormone called cholecystokinin (CCK). CCK is one of the body chemicals that is normally released to tell the brain that we have had enough to eat, that we are "full."

If this chemical is released early enough, you can eat less without having hunger pangs. If you eat less, but eat "smart," you will have an adequate supply of nutrients and will be able to burn body fat for energy instead of just storing food away.

L–phenylalanine needs vitamins to be effective, particularly vitamin C and vitamin B–6 (pyrodoxine). It is important to be taking a good multiple vitamin/mineral formula when you diet. More about vitamins and any cautions later on.

Additional benefits from L–phenylalanine include help in the production of natural epinephrine, a hormone manufactured by the adrenal glands, useful as a body stimulant, and thyroxine, a hormone needed to regulate the metabolic rate of the body. You need help in the production of the natural hormone that raises the metabolic rate of your body. Well, here it is. The metabolic rate governs the pace at which the body operates and the speed with which it burns fat. A sluggish rate burns fat more slowly.

L–phenylalanine also plays an important part in overcoming the desire to eat when you are feeling "blue."

There are many over–the–counter drugs available to help suppress your appetite. Some of these widely advertised products contain a substance that sounds like L–phenylalanine but isn't. It's called phenylpropanolamine (PPA). It works by causing the release of noradrenaline in the brain the same way that L–phenylalanine does.

It doesn't trick the brain into making more of the noradrenaline, however, so it loses its ability in a very short span of time.

L–phenylalanine will work each time you use it. You do not lose the effectiveness after a few weeks.

Availability: Most health food stores and drugstores.

Dosage: *100 to 500 mg* with about 250 mg vitamin C, and 25 to 50 mg vitamin B–6 or a multivitamin and mineral supplement that contains both, at bedtime.

100 to 500 mg with vitamins in the morning before breakfast with a full glass of water. If the exciting quality of the amino acid should interfere with sleep, either reduce the dose or eliminate the nighttime dose.

You may want to take L–phenylalanine before lunch and supper as well if you want to speed up the weight–loss process; however, as soon as you reach your desired weight, reduce the dosage to 100 to 500 mg at night or in the morning, to help you maintain your weight.

Amino acids are natural substances, but once you are satisfied with your condition, it's best to return the control over neurotransmitters to your body.

You should be able to then remain at your best weight through appetite control and exercise.

If, however, you should have to resort to the use of amino acids again, you can do so with the same safety as before.

Should I See a Doctor Before I Go on a Diet?

It's always a good idea to go to your nutrition–oriented doctor before you begin any diet, whether you're going to use the natural substances in this book, or any other weight–loss method.

Your doctor can advise you about exercise and your present physical condition, when to exercise, and how strenuous the exercise routine should be.

He or she can also advise when to increase the amount and the duration of the program.

The doctor, knowing your medical history can also advise the use of amino acids or advise against the use, since there are certain very rare cases where one or more of these food substances should be avoided in the amount here suggested. (See chapter on Contraindications.)

On the whole, amino acids are completely safe for the vast majority of people, but it pays to be cautious if you suffer from certain genetic conditions.

When Should I Avoid Using L–phenylalanine?

- If you suffer from high blood pressure. A few sensitive individuals may experience a rise in pressure even at the low doses suggested.
- If you suffer from the genetic disease phenylketonuria (PKU).
- If your doctor has prescribed a monoamine oxidase (MAO) inhibitor.

Great! I Do Have a Bit of High Blood Pressure Because I Am Overweight. First You Tell Me the Good News; Then You Tell Me I Can't Use It!

Maybe you can't use L–phenylalanine, but you *can* use something else.

L–tryosine

Here's another essential amino acid with all of the brain–changing qualities of L–phenylalanine, but without the blood–pressure–raising side effect some sensitive people experience. Incidentally, not all people with high blood pressure have to avoid using L–phenylalanine. Most people will *not* find that it affects their pressure. I only bring it up to make sure that you will monitor your pressure if you suspect some deviation. Your doctor can help you make a decision by teaching you to use a blood pressure device so you can test yourself at home.

Why Not Just Use L–tyrosine in the First Place?

While L–tyrosine will produce the same brain chemicals as L–phenylalanine (L–tyrosine→noradrenaline→dopamine), it may not influence the production of CCK in the intestine. However, it decreases appetite, helps overcome the "blues," improves mental alertness and ambition, and leads to a more positive outlook on life.

L–tyrosine is also found naturally in meat, dairy products, and eggs. Although it is not an essential amino acid, since it can be manufactured (with difficulty) in the body, it is one of the more important food factors concerned with brain chemistry.

Availability: Most health food stores and drugstores.

Dosage: 100 to 500 mg with about 250 mg vitamin C, and 25 to 50 mg vitamin B–6, or a vitamin and mineral supplement that contains both, at bedtime or before breakfast.

Begin with the smaller dose of L–tyrosine and slowly increase it until you begin to feel the effect on your appetite. You may want to raise or lower the dose at your pleasure.

Although L–tyrosine usually has no effect on blood pressure, it is wise to monitor its use anyway. Anybody can have an unusual reaction to anything—even to water!

The Food and Drug Administration (FDA) has recognized both L–phenylalanine and L–tyrosine as nutrients only, and has not approved them as agents against obesity or for any activity other than as a food supplement.

As with any of the amino acids, please read the chapter on contra-indications!

L–glutamine

Although nature is almost always right, sometimes it makes an error. It put the brain in a place in the body that appeared to be the safest, surrounded by the hard, bony skull. Then, it guarded the brain with a barrier that's supposed to block the entrance of any harmful substance. However, for some reason, *this system blocked the entrance of one of the two substances that the brain eats!*

The brain consumes glucose and glutamic acid for energy. Without these high–energy foods, the brain would starve to death. Glutamic acid and glucose (blood sugar) are the foods the brain needs and wants.

So, when the brain is hungry and in need of nutrients, it sends messages to the stomach that increase the appetite for food and increase desire for sweets that contain sugar in their most digestible form. By doing this, the hungry brain can wreck the most careful diet.

That's What Happened to Me Four Diets Ago!

It happens to lots of people—an uncontrollable urge to gorge on candy or some other sweet.

It's really that the brain is hungry and needs something to munch on.

How Can I Fight It?

That's the story of a relative to glutamic acid called L–glutamine.

Through nutritional magic and by the use of L–glutamine, we can feed the brain and quiet its craving for sweets.

L–glutamine is the amide form of glutamic acid. Because L–glutamine can cross the brain barrier easily, and the brain can take it and quickly convert it into glutamic acid, if you take L–glutamine in supplemental form the brain will be able to satisfy its hunger more easily.

You can take large amounts of glutamic acid and get only a trivial rise of glutamic acid in the brain, but moderate amounts of L–glutamine produces a marked elevation of glutamic acid!

Glutamic acid is not made into brain chemicals called neurotransmitters, as are some of the amino acids, nor is glutamic acid incorporated into the protein structure of the brain.

Glutamic acid has two major functions. It serves primarily as a fuel for the brain's operation, and serves as a buffer against excess ammonia.

The relationship of glutamic acid to glucose (blood sugar) goes beyond the brain–fuel interrelationship. The brain can store only a small amount of glucose. Therefore, the brain is very dependent on the second–to–second supply of blood sugar. This may explain dizziness and other nervous symptoms that accompany hypoglycemia (low blood sugar).

The gray matter in the brain converts glutamic acid to a special compound that helps to regulate brain cell activity. Thus, a shortage of L–glutamine in the diet, and of glutamic acid in the brain, can result in brain damage due to excess ammonia or a brain that cannot get into "high gear."

Where Can I Get L–glutamine and How Much Do I Take?

Availability: Most health food stores and drugstores. Do not buy glutamic acid.

Dosage: If you have an "irresistible" craving for sweets, L–glutamine can help you control it. According to Dr. H. L. Newbold, if you want to take L–glutamine to lift your spirits, begin with a 200 mg capsule or tablet three times a day for one week. Then increase the dose to two capsules or tablets three times a day for one week.

If you feel more alert, more energetic, and have lost your craving for sweets, you can then experiment with the amount of L–glutamine you take until you find the best level for you.

Alcoholism Can Be Brought on by the Anxiety of Dieting

Dieting is stressful!

Some people who are not necessarily fond of alcohol may find that they resort to drinking a lot more than usual in an effort to control the stress they feel.

Also, since alcohol is metabolized very quickly, it is converted to brain fuel, and during your diet your brain can feel hungry and ask for a drink. If you answer its request and continue to do so you can do more than just wreck your diet program.

Dr. Roger Williams, along with his colleagues at the Clayton Foundation for Research at the University of Texas, made the vital discovery that not only did L–glutamine protect against the poisonous effects of alcohol; it also controlled or stopped completely the craving for it.

L–glutamine is a versatile amino acid that can contribute to your diet program if, on your way to your best weight level, you suffer from any of the problems described.

Cholecystokinin (CCK)

This wonder substance for no–effort weight loss was envisioned as long ago as 1910, when Pavlov suggested that appetite was somehow regulated by signals sent from the stomach to the hypothalamus in the brain.

Until Pavlov brought this concept into being, no one considered how we stop eating. The stomach is a relatively small sack, but it can expand. People assumed that when it was full we felt physically satisfied and just stopped shoveling in food. But some people never feel satisfied and just eat and snack the whole day through; so, it's not just the physical feeling that controls food intake volume.

Pavlov considered that there must be some kind of chemical released at the ingestion point (the stomach) that was able to travel through the blood stream to the brain, so that the brain would issue the command to cease and desist!

In 1980, two noted scientists, G. P. Smith and J. Gibbs, collaborated on the following statement. "Our ignorance about mechanisms for post–prandial satiety is total; no one knows what mechanism(s) terminate any meal in any organism at any time."

In other words, the medical and nutritional establishment still doesn't understand fully how and why our bodies know when we have taken in enough food to satisfy our energy needs.

The literature on satiety mechanisms supports the idea that a number of different pathways are required to let the brain know when to close our mouths.

That's one of the problems.

If your body chooses a slow passageway to tell the brain, which then uses a slow passageway to tell the mouth to stop eating, another 2,000 calories can be ingested in the interim!

It would be naive to accept the fact that a single substance, in some manner, would be able to carry the entire burden, but there was a great deal of interest shown in a substance called cholecystokinin (CCK) when it elicited satiety in a form of obese rats.

Rats, given injections of CCK, will sit before a bowl of their favorite food and not eat. Although they have not touched food for hours, they are convinced that they have eaten a full meal. In some cases, with repeated injections of CCK, they will refuse food even to the point of starving themselves to death!

However, appetite, food, and satiety are very complicated subjects. If CCK were only found in the stomach, it might have been isolated much earlier, but CCK occurs in large amounts in almost all regions of the central nervous system and appears to be an active neurotransmitter. Only after much careful observation was it discovered that the CCK peptides may act differently at different sites in the body and play different roles.

Experiments have now shown that CCK can act in the bloodstream, the same way a hormone does, as well as in the nerves as a neurotransmitter.

In Spite of What My Relatives Think, I'm Not a Rat

Humans and rats have relatively similar digestive systems. What affects a rat's digestion will usually have the same result with a human.

The difficulty with sticking to a low–calorie diet is feeling completely satisfied at the end of a meal. If satiety is not reached, the compulsion to snack can lead to excess caloric intake.

Also, diets are stressful, and stress–induced eating has long been recognized in wild animals and in humans. Psychological stress can produce a number of behavioral abnormalities, and overeating is one of them.

Enter CCK

Presumably, if CCK could be taken before meals, it would reach the stomach and send a signal to the brain that the body had taken in enough food.

Take CCK just before meals. By doing this, there should still be time for you to eat enough to keep your body healthy and happy. Then the false signal will be sent to your brain that you are "stuffed," and any chance for you to gorge yourself will be over for that meal.

CCK Clinical Weight–loss Study

A four–week clinical weight–loss study was conduced using CCK tablets. The study was a random placebo–controlled study using thirty–nine individuals consisting of 28 percent male subjects. The individuals ranged in age from eighteen to sixty–six. The patients met the requirements set forth by 21 CFR Part 357 for obese patients. This requirement dictates that weight–loss participants be a minimum of 15 percent overweight when compared to the height and weight standards set forth by the 1983 Metropolitan Life Insurance Company. The patients were weighed in weekly at the same time to minimize weight fluctuations other than those created by the diet study. Each patient was given a hospital–formulated diet of 1200 to 1400 calories per day and an oral diet supplement consisting of a placebo or CCK.

The dosage was two tablets taken before each meal and at mid–evening. The patients receiving the CCK diet supplement lost an average of 12.05 pounds per each patient, over the four weeks, as compared to the placebo group which averaged a loss of 2.15 pounds each for the same time period. CCK greatly surpasses the requirements for a "clinically effective" weight–loss product as defined by 21 *Code of Federal Regulations* Part 357.

Those patients who were given CCK lost up to 23 pounds in the four–week period. Eighty percent of these patients had a significant weight loss.

The control group—who were not given CCK—lost only a few pounds, despite their diet.

The CCK Clinical Weight Loss Study concludes that CCK is an extremely effective weight–loss product that surpasses government standards for products of this category.

In addition, the product was well–liked by the participants of the study, many volunteering testimonials on its behalf.

In a paper entitled "Immunochemical Studies on Cholecystokinin," Jen F. Rehfeld of the Institute of Medical Biochemistry, University of Aarhus, Denmark, states that the highest level of naturally occurring CCK is in brain tissues.

It is present in brain tissue at a level of 925 picomoles per gm of wet tissue. This calculates to a level of 62 picomoles of active supplement.

CCK has been found to exert the satiety effect in levels as low as 0.1 picomoles per ml.

CCK exists in a precursor form of thirty–three amino acids. The tryptic cleavage of CCK 33 to CCK 8 is necessary to activate the peptide. CCK exerts its putative effect in the stomach. CCK is heat– and acid–stable.

The body is stimulated to produce CCK by several entities: acid, fatty acids, amino acids, proteoses.

CCK's site of action is in the stomach. The CCK in supplement form is broken down in the stomach by the enzyme–acid conditions.

Thus, orally supplied CCK could survive in the stomach environment and, in fact, be activated by the acid–enzyme condition.

The Problem

Because CCK is a natural substance, but not considered to be a nutritional supplement, the FDA ordered it to be pulled from the market.

Pharmaceutical companies will not go through all of the testing procedures because they can't patent it.

So why did I bother to write about it?

One reason is that some pharmaceutical companies will modify it and offer it for sale on prescription. If it is available it will probably be one of the few substances that will help the obese person. You'll have you ask your nutrition–oriented physician to watch for it.

The other reason is that you may still be able to find it in some weight–reducing formulas at your health food store. If you do locate one of these, follow manufacturer's instructions.

Dehydroepiandrosterone (DHEA)

A little–known hormone with an almost unpronounceable name, dehydroepiandrosterone (DHEA), may be the answer to a dieter's prayer. It can be a fountain of youth and miracle weight reducer.

Imagine Being Able to Lose Weight without Altering Your Diet

This may be the result gathered from experiments begun by a research biochemist at Temple University's Fels Research Institute in Philadelphia.

Dr. Arthur G. Schwartz holds a doctorate in microbiology from Harvard University and post–doctoral fellowships at both Oxford University and the Albert Einstein College of Medicine in New York City. He recently discovered that a particular hormone (DHEA) is produced in the body in very large quantities up until the mid–20s, and then begins decreasing at a steady rate as the body ages.

It appears that this Concentrated Fat–Burner blocks an enzyme that the body uses to produce glucose. If the body can't process the sugar, it can't store it either.

The way this Concentrated Fat–Burner works, proposed by Dr. Schwartz, is that it increases the body's ability to transform food directly into energy.

This enables the body to 'burn off' old excess fat—and to prevent new fat from accumulating in the first place.

Schwartz's controlled experiments confirmed that DHEA will cause obese mice to lose weight even as they continue eating their regular menu and without the addition of any appetite–controlling substances.

The mice eat normally. *It's just that the calories are then converted to heat rather than fat, thereby allowing the animals to lose weight!*

DHEA inhibits an enzyme called NAPDH (G–6–PDH) that is used by the body to manufacture fatty acids, which then become fat in the body. If the action of NAPDH is restrained, less fat is created. The chart that follows illustrates this action.

Other research suggests that DHEA may have stress–reducing properties as well as weight–reducing properties.

Dr. Norman Applezweig, a biochemist, dreams that DHEA may reduce the diseases of aging and perhaps even prolong life. Applezweig says that he believes that DHEA slows down hormones that cause premature–aging factors in the body, thereby slowing down the aging process itself.

Now for the Bad News

DHEA is hard to find in the marketplace!

The pharmaceutical industry is the logical place to raise money for research and development of DHEA. Extremely large sums of money are needed to prepare a substance to pass the FDA's tests for public safety, and many years of double–blind and other studies must be finished and presented before a product can reach the market.

Because DHEA is a natural hormone whose medical uses have already been reported and publicized, *it cannot be patented.* However promising, it would be foolish to spend the millions of dollars necessary for testing if the company testing could not recoup its investment and make a profit.

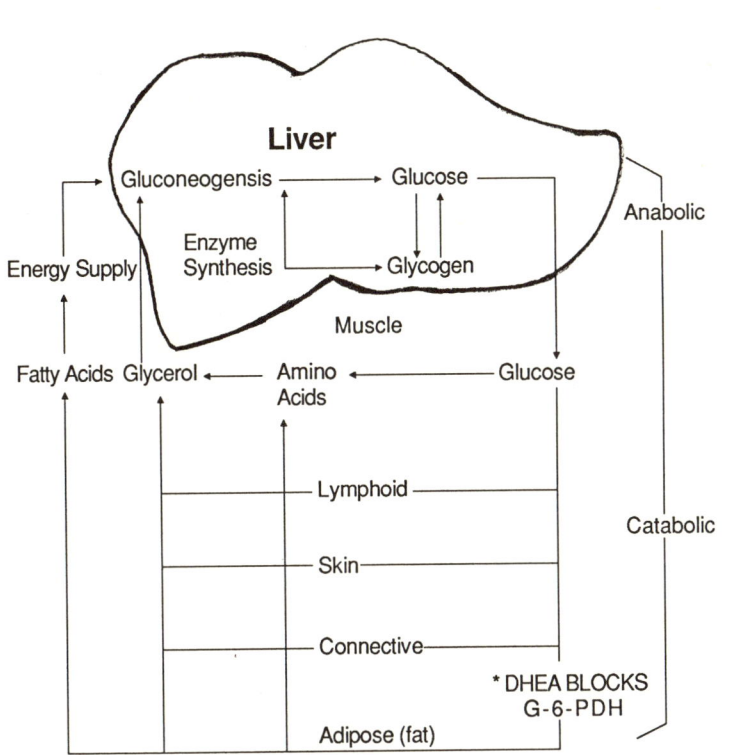

Liver

Gluconeogensis — → Glucose

Enzyme
Synthesis

Energy Supply

Glycogen

Anabolic

Muscle

Fatty Acids Glycerol ←— Amino ←——— Glucose
Acids

——— Lymphoid ———

—— Skin——

——— Connective———

* DHEA BLOCKS
G-6-PDH

Adipose (fat)

Catabolic

The Chemistry & Functions of the Hormones

And a Bit of Good News

Nature never concentrates all of its resources in one species. There is a member of the vegetable kingdom, the same Mexican yam that provided the steroids for the first birth control pill, that appears to be an abundant source of DHEA.

It is not approved by the FDA, even as a nutritional supplement, but it has been incorporated into a few weight–reducing formulas available at some health food stores.

You'll have to a be a detective and read labels carefully, but with perseverance and by asking questions you can find DHEA.

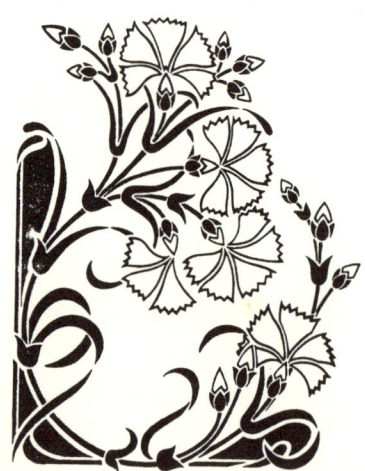

The Fat–Burners

Fats are the most concentrated energy source in the diet. When they are "burned" (combined with oxygen), they enable the body to function on all levels. There are many natural substances to "burn off" fat.

The more efficient the burning, the more energy is released, and the more fat is used up.

Therefore, if obesity is being fostered by inefficiency in the fat–burning mechanism, and that can be corrected easily with a dietary supplement, then a program of exercise, reduced caloric intake, and the use of that supplement should result in a new, slim person.

Coenzyme Q–10

Coenzyme Q–10, also known as ubiquinone (named after the word *ubiquitous*, which means "found everywhere," because it is present in almost every cell in the body), has a structure similar to that of vitamin K.

It is part of the biochemical pathway from which adenosine triphosphate (ATP) and metabolic energy are derived to run individual cells and the entire body.

Since most cellular functions are dependent on the availability of energy, Coenzyme Q–10 is essential for the health of all human tissues and organs. Although it can be manufactured in the body, deficiencies of the substance have been reported in a wide range of conditions, including obesity.

The tendency to become overweight may be associated in some cases with a certain metabolic makeup that results in decreased heat production. Many scientists now believe that most people do not gain weight because they eat too much. Instead, they gain weight because their bodies work against their efforts to diet—putting the pounds in storage rather than burning them.

Human subjects with a family history of obesity have a 50 percent reduction in their thermogenic response to meals, suggesting the existence of an hereditary defect in energy production.

Since coenzyme Q–10 is an essential cofactor for energy production, *it is possible that a deficiency is a contributing cause of obesity.*

During tests, serum coenzyme Q–10 levels were found to be low in 52 percent of the obese subjects tests. When they were given 100 mg of coenzyme Q–10, along with a calorie–restricted diet, there was a mean weight loss of thirty pounds in eight weeks.

This study suggests that about half of obese people may be deficient in coenzyme Q–10, and that treatment accelerates weight loss during a low–calorie diet.

Availability: If you need it, if you have a history of fat in the family, you can find coenzyme Q–10 in health food stores and drugstores.

Dosage: Coenzyme Q–10 comes in 10 mg capsules or tablets. Try taking one capsule three times a day and vary the dose until you find the most appropriate dose for you. Usually two capsules three times a day is the top dosage for most people.

How about Safety?

Coenzyme Q–10 is generally well–tolerated, and no serious adverse effects have been reported. However, it is not recommended during pregnancy and lactation, or in cases of known hypersensitivity. The FDA considers it to be only a food supplement, and it is not recognized for weight control.

Cytochrome C

One of the great difficulties dieters have to contend with is fatigue. However, fatigue and diet no longer have to be associated if a simple combination of amino acids and iron are part of your diet program.

Called cytochrome C, this newly–discovered miracle is available without a prescription at your health food store or at most drugstores.

What Does It Do?

Every cell has to breathe. Cells don't have lungs the way we do, but they need oxygen in order to live and work. The cells have a little engine called the mitochrondria, which also needs oxygen to burn for energy. If cells don't have enough oxygen, you feel fatigue. Cytochrome C increases the amount of oxygen carried to and exchanged with the cells.

What Happens if There Is Insufficient Oxygen?

Have you ever started to exercise and had to stop because your muscles began to cramp and burn? You may have thought it was because you were out of shape, but your exercise time (very important if you want to burn off fat and lose weight) can be improved if you supplement with cytochrome C.

When you exercise, the various cells involved must have oxygen to burn. This is called aerobic respiration. If there is not enough oxygen brought to the cells, the cells can switch over to another method of obtaining energy called anaerobic (without oxygen).

What's So Bad about That if It Provides Energy?

The anaerobic method (without oxygen) produces lactic acid, which causes muscles to burn. The lactic acid can remain in the muscles and case soreness the next day.

This lack of cytochrome C could explain why some people tire so easily no matter how little they exercise. The lactic acid build–up will cut down on endurance. A trained athlete would have higher levels of cytochrome C in the body than the average person, but you can raise your levels of this important substance to athletic levels without vigorous and boring training procedures by taking cytochrome C as a supplement.

You Wouldn't Call Cytochrome C a Diet Pill?

Not by itself.

Exercise speeds weight loss, but if exercise hurts, you won't continue it for any length of time. So, as far as exercise is concerned, cytochrome C is a diet pill. Also, since it helps the body burn fats more efficiently, it helps rid the body of fat that would otherwise be stored away in great lumps under the skin.

A decrease in the amount of food intake can deplete the body of a certain amount of energy and promote a feeling of lassitude. This lack of energy can influence the desire to "bend" the diet rigors and snack on a sugary food.

While the use of a high–potency vitamin/mineral supplement can help to ward off this tired feeling, there are also some other nutritional aids to help increase muscle performance and endurance, and to help keep the energy level more or less constant.

A detailed survey of the literature over the past decade reveals a large body of work done on the relationship of the cytochromes to an increase in performance.

Since cytochrome C is a major link in the respiratory chain, and muscle performance is dependent on aerobic respiration, cytochrome C appears to be an obvious aid to the dieter.

Cytochrome C is a simple chemical compound composed of a series of amino acids and iron, found naturally in the body. This compound acts as a carrier of oxygen to the mitochondria, which are the cellular furnaces that feed energy to the individual cell. The energy allows the muscles to work. The more cytochrome C available, the more readily the muscles expand and contract before fatigue sets in.

When diet limits the amount of cytochrome C that will be manufactured in the body, supplemental use of this substance can help ward off the fatigue which might normally hinder the dieter.

Availability: Cytochrome C is often found in energy formulas at health food stores and drugstores. It is also available in tablet form.

Dosage: If you purchase cytochrome C in an energy mix, follow manufacturer's directions. Otherwise, two 250 mg tablets in the morning are enough for the average dieter. If your doctor advises a strenuous exercise program, along with a cut in calories, you might want to take one more in the afternoon.

Gamma–cryzanol (GO)

Many dieters are taking a page from the body–beautiful people. Weight lifters who want to keep their muscles up and their fat down have found a white powder called gamma–cryzanol, extracted from rice bran oil. If you want to develop a slim, strong, athletic–looking figure, this may be your best—and easiest—bet.

It increases lean body mass, decreases fatty tissue, helps fight the energy loss brought on by dieting, and may help relieve the stress symptoms that accompany menopause.

Why Haven't I Heard about Gamma–cryzanol Before?

Although it was discovered more than thirty years ago by a Japanese researcher, it only recently came to the attention of body builders trying to get more out of their workouts. They found that gamma–cryzanol (called GO) was an ergogenic aid.

What's an Ergogenic Aid?

It's any work–enhancing energy–producing substance that can be used to effectively improve performance, if taken for competition purposes. It also fights the energy drain of dieting.

How Does It Work?

Although its exact method of operation is still unknown, it probably works on the hypothalamus in the brain, which has direct contact with the central nervous system. Through its control of the pituitary gland, the hypothalamus governs a number of your body's automatic functions, including temperature control, water balance, and hormonal regulation. Those hormones include the sex hormones—testosterone in the male and estrogen in the female.

It appears that GO may increase testosterone production. This may be the reason for an increase in lean body mass that researchers have observed when laboratory animals were fed a diet supplemented with this nutrient.

Researchers have also observed that fatty tissue appears to decrease when GO is used as a supplement in conjunction with controlled caloric intake and an exercise program.

What Else Does It Do?

It might benefit women in other ways besides dieting. There have been controlled experiments in which GO has been administered to women and brought about a blessed reduction of the painful symptoms of menopause—without the slightest need for hormones or drugs.

GO also has a life–saving effect on another front.

Free radicals, extremely active particles generated in the body, can penetrate body cells and cause intense damage. Free radicals have been called one of the causes of degenerative diseases and one of the causes of the signs of aging.

GO acts as an antioxidant, meaning it helps to neutralize those chemical particles before they can do damage. The exercise you do to help you lose weight can contribute to the production of these free radicals, but that doesn't mean you shouldn't exercise. It does mean you should use the protective nutrients nature has provided to keep your body healthy.

GO, vitamin E, selenium, vitamin A, vitamin C, and cysteine, among other nutritional supplements, will help to counter any free radicals from within or from without, which is another good reason to take a strong multi–vitamin and mineral supplement while you are on your diet, and after as well.

There are some formulas on the market that combine GO with some of the other antioxidant and protective nutrients.

Availability: Found in health food stores. Some drugstores also carry it.

Dosage: If you do normal exercise, take 5 mg daily. If you do heavy exercise, you can take up to 15 mg daily.

The FDA has not authorized GO as anything but a nutritional supplement.

Phosphosugar

This compound is sugar and phosphorus combined. It is a basic source of energy to the body. For phosphorus to be an energy source, it must be linked to sugar. For sugar to be metabolized and be an energy source, it must be linked to phosphorus.

How Does the Body Use This Compound for Energy?

It is an intermediate block of the compound adenosine triphosphate (ATP), which is the most important substance of cellular energy. The TP stands for "triphosphate"—three phosphates (phosphorus). When the body requires energy, it splits the three–phosphate group into a one–phosphate and a two–phosphate. When the molecule is split (just like when an atom is split for atomic power), useful metabolid energy is re-leased.

Where Does the Body Find a Use for This Energy?

Whenever any body function occurs, energy is required. Every body cell must have energy to live and carry on its work. Without phospho-sugar, the energy release would not be possible.

What Does It Have To Do with My Diet?

Most dieters go on a low–carbohydrate diet. This interferes with the amount of energy the body is capable of producing. As the energy level decreases, so does the ability to concentrate, exercise, and do work of any sort. The brain, feeling overly tired, sends out the command to eat more carbohydrates, thereby interfering with the continuation of the diet.

Under normal conditions, persons eating a well–balanced diet will derive phosphosugar from their food sources. These will be linked with natural sugars, which the body converts to metabolic energy. However, dieters, by reducing carbohydrate intake, will deplete themselves of their carbohydrate and fat reserves.

This is done on purpose, because this is one way to lose pounds, and why go on a diet if not to lose weight?

When carried to an extreme, carbohydrate reduction forces the body to break down amino acids for energy. If the intake of protein is also in-adequate, the body may break down its own protein, including the protein that goes to make up the muscles.

If the intake of phosphorus is inadequate, the body may even rob the bones of their phosphorus content.

Therefore, your diet must consist of at least one meal a day contain-ing adequate amounts of protein, plus fresh vegetables to prevent breakdown of protein.

Use of Phosphosugar

This substance is not fattening because the sugars are glucose and fructose (monosaccharides). Glucose is the primary source of energy for humans. The excess over what the body uses for energy is not turned into fat. Glucose is not metabolized unless it is first bound to phosphorus.

Fructose is a fruit sugar that produces glycogen and maintains nor-mal content of glucose in the blood. In the liver, it may be converted into glycogen, which in turn may be converted into glucose.

Phosphosugar contains the ingredients needed by the body to make ATP, which fuels your cells.

Availability: This is another product that may be difficult to find, since all health food stores do not stock it. However, if you search and ask around you will be able to locate it.

Dosage: When you locate it, follow manufacturer's directions. Usually you would use it twice a day, say before breakfast and before lunch. It comes in small packets, should be mixed with a citrus juice. It has a slightly bitter taste, even though it sounds as if it ought to be sweet. The FDA has not approved this product as a diet aid.

Carnitine

L–carnitine is the fat–burner that works at your body's deepest level— without any help from your will power!

There are many preparations on the market that say they will help you lose weight. Many of them are based on a protein formula supplemented by vitamins and minerals. They are to be used as substitutes for at least two of your regular meals, and, to some extent, they do help some of us lose a few pounds. However, people who use these proteins and vitamins still complain they feel hungry after they have taken their meal substitute.

That's no way to feel when you're on a diet, especially when there are so many tempting foods around.

People feeling hungry have resorted to having their jaws wired shut! Others have had their stomachs surgically restricted so they could feel full after a tiny meal.

There has to be a better way!

What about a pill that would quiet your appetite and help you to lose weight at the same time? A natural substance with a good safety record to help you turn down a cookie and feel good about yourself. Does it exist? I think so.

It's called L–carnitine and it's part of the amino family. The same family that gives you L–phenylalanine, L–tyrosine, and so on.

We owe a lot to that family. And, here's another debt.

Is L–carnitine Something New?

No!

It was discovered in 1907, but its critical role in the body was not recognized for fifty years, and it wasn't until 1973 that doctors first recognized that people could have a carnitine deficiency.

Up until then, doctors and nutritionists assumed that the body would make enough carnitine if there were not enough in the diet.

L–carnitine is not considered an essential nutrient because it can be manufactured in the liver of humans from the amino acids lysine and methionine, provided that there are sufficient quantities of vitamins B–3, B–6, and C present at the same time. However, recent research indicates that L–carnitine plays an *important role in converting stored body fat into energy.*

It is also important in controlling hypoglycemia, energizing the heart, reducing the effects of angina attacks, and is beneficial to patients suffering from diabetes, liver disease, or kidney disease.

How Does L–carnitine Burn Fat?

Think about the carburetor in your car, how it functions, and what it does. In cars, the carburetor regulates the flow of fuel (gasoline) into the engine. The flow of fuel determines how much is burned to produce the power necessary to run the car.

In the body, in each of the billions of cells, there is a miniature engine that resembles the engine in a car. The engine is called the mitochrondrion; it burns fat for energy.

But the fat cannot get into the fuel line by itself. It needs something to ferry it through the wall of the mitochondrion.

Scientists discovered that the inner wall of the mitochondrion contains an enzyme called carnitine acyltransferase, which transfers a molecule of fat to carnitine, linking the two together. Then, although the fat molecule alone cannot enter the engine to be burned, once it is linked to carnitine it passes without any trouble at all.

Therefore, carnitine accelerates the rate at which the body burns fat. *The more fat that is burned—the less you have to carry around with you.*

To put it another way, without a sufficient supply of carnitine you wouldn't have the energy to turn the pages in this book!

The more you take of carnitine, the more fat your body can burn, and the more energy you get from your body.

When your body has an excess of fat, it stores it in the fat cells and also in the liver. The condition known as "fatty liver" may be due to the body's inability to manufacture enough carnitine.

Is it any wonder that nutritionists are excited about this substance?

How Else Does Carnitine Help in Weight Reduction?

You've heard of "Brown Fat," the fat tissue that helps us acclimate to cold temperatures and is thought to help determine how much of the food we eat is burned for heat and how much is converted to stored body fat. Well, L–carnitine plays a vital role in the production of that heat.

Once again, the more L–carnitine is available, the more fat is burned off to keep the temperature of the body constant. That's why you can lose weight in the summer, sitting around in your shorts watching television, if you lower the air conditioner to keep the room at 72 degrees. The Brown Fat will burn White Fat to keep you at your standard 98.6 degrees.

The engines in the body that use L–carnitine as a substrate are critical to energy production. In the absence of L–carnitine, large fat molecules cannot be burned. They build up in the blood stream as fats and triglycerides. L–carnitine–deficient persons often have bouts of hypoglycemia (low blood sugar levels), with a nagging feeling of lassitude and severe lack of energy.

Poor Weight–loss Diets Can Be a Danger

Some people, desperate to lose weight, sometimes use bad judgment when going on a diet. They may choose an all–protein diet, with the possibility of running into "acid blood" conditions. The problem is called "ketosis," and when uncontrolled, can be life–threatening. Even when not life–threatening, ketosis causes the loss of important minerals such as potassium, calcium, and magnesium.

L–carnitine prevents ketones from accumulating. If your doctor suggests a protein diet (may be helpful for a short time under medical supervision), then ask about L–carnitine. Don't be afraid to ask. It's your body!

L–carnitine and the Heart

Can there be a pill to help you lose weight that's also good for your heart?

Say hello to L–carnitine once more.

The heart produces most of its energy from fats, thus it is dependent on L–carnitine. A deficiency causes extreme metabolic impairment to heart tissue.

On the other hand, supplements of L–carnitine have proved to be beneficial to heart patients. They have increased the exercise endurance, lowered the exercise heart rate, extended the exercise time, reduced the number of angina attacks and nitroglycerine consumption.

How About L–carnitine and Athletes?

Evidence mounts up that L–carnitine supplementation produces the efficient fat–burning you want during prolonged exercise. It has been found to be even more important because the level of fat utilization for muscle energy rises during the exercise period. Also that it prevents muscle fatigue, and increases tolerance to stress.

A study headed by Dr. Kevin Pfefferle, at the University of Wyoming, tested for percent body fat, exercise performance, and pulse recovery on wrestlers and distance runners. They were given a daily dose of L–carnitine, twice daily. Not only was there a confirmed loss of body fat—but better total pulse recovery from these strenuous exercises.

Are There Dietary Sources of L–carnitine?

The major sources are meat and dairy products. There is little or no L–carnitine in fruits and vegetables. The amount found in food may be enough for normal usage, but not enough for weight loss.

Availability: In health food stores and drugstores. It can be purchased alone or in combination with other weight–loss substances.

Dosage: It may be taken in a 250 mg tablet twice daily; however, if there is any evidence of allergy (people can be allergic to anything, even water) the use of L–carnitine alone should be discontinued and the use of a combination with other substances should be considered.

The FDA does not consider L–carnitine to be anything but a food supplement.

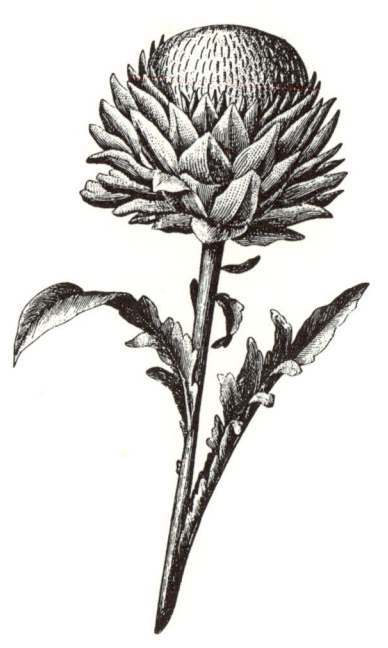

Trade In Fat for Muscle

For years all you've been told is "the only way to lose weight is to eat less."

Millions of people set about to eat less and hope to get thin. Once they get thin they try to stay thin.

But if dieting is considered to be the only "cure" for obesity, then it's a pretty bad cure, with a terrible success rate!

Most people who diet either don't lose the weight they want to lose or, if they do lose weight, they put it back in a very short time.

A lot of their diet problems rest with Diet Panic and Diet Stress, but we went into that earlier in the book. Just as soon as you go on that stringent weight–loss, calorie–cutting diet, panic and stress wake up and haunt you.

Dieting is an Unscientific Way to Lose Weight!

It is based on the puritanical belief that the "overindulgence" that leads to fat must be punished by the pain of such dieting.

A little like punishing you because you indulge in sex! It's fun to eat and it's satisfying.

Another reason dieting is the usual medical answer to obesity is that no doctor has come up with any other kind of cure.

However, a Cure for Obesity May Be Just around the Corner

About ten years ago, give or take, researchers discovered the presence of a special hormone in the human body. They named it "Human Growth Hormone" (HGH).

What was curious about this substance is that when it was given to animals, they were able to eat huge amounts of food without growing fat. In fact, they ended up in better physical condition than before they began the test.

Someone began to speculate about friends of theirs—lean, hungry, thin people who eat huge amounts of food but seldom vary their weight more than a couple of pounds either way. Could their fat–burning powers be due to HGH?

When they investigated further, they discovered that the HGH levels in lean people were higher than the HGH levels in obese people.

According to Pearson and Shaw, in their book *Life Extension*, "Growth hormone causes one to put on muscle and burn fat. Everyone knows that most teenagers eat like horses without becoming obese, even if they are sedentary. A middle–aged person eating the same food and getting the same exercise will usually become fat. The higher growth hormone levels in teenagers have a great deal to do with the difference."

How Does It Work Its Miracle?

HGH is stored in the pituitary gland in all healthy people. One of its purposes is to make sure that during the growing years, fat can be converted into fuel and into muscle tissue to serve the needs of the growing body.

So, Why Does It Stop Working for Me?

Don't feel slighted, it stops for most people.

As we age, the release of HGH slows down, and, by the age of thirty (not old by any means), the flow has virtually ceased.

Why?

We don't have a definite answer. We do know that HGH is still manufactured and still stored in the pituitary gland. Some people speculate that the flow of HGH is cut off as a protection to older people. Perhaps older people need the extra amount of fat to stay warm, and as extra fuel in case there is a shortage of food.

Remember, this body system was set up a long time ago to help people survive in caves, not in today's world, where homes are heated by burning gas or oil, and where there is a supermarket or shopping mall just around the corner.

But when you diet (remember that the body thinks in terms of famine), the body does not respond by released HGH. It does just the opposite.

The more you starve yourself, the more your body fights you!

O.K., What Do I Have To Do?

Nutritional magic!

Bypass the diet and go directly to HGH release.

It was established in the mid–seventies that injections of certain amino acids could trigger release of HGH.

Watch out—injections mean doctors, bills, prescriptions. Just what I want you to avoid. So why have I included HGH in this book? *Because we've traded in the needle for some pills!*

In June of 1982, Pearson and Shaw said, "The amino acids L–arginine and L–ornithine, taken on an empty stomach at bedtime, cause growth hormone release. These can easily make a normal 65–year–old's growth hormone levels resemble those of a teenager."

L–arginine and L–ornithine work together to stimulate the release of growth hormones from the pituitary gland in the brain.

This is probably why L–arginine and L–ornithine have been effective in cases of trauma and in general debility where the immune system has been weakened. By toning the entire system, they can reduce recovery time from many abnormalities and promote wound healing.

Human Growth Hormone does many things in the body. It can:

- increase the basal metabolic rate and burn off fat during sleep;
- help build attractive muscle tissue by enhancing protein synthesis at the same time it burns off White Fat;
- repair tendons and ligaments;
- improve the immune response;
- stimulate the thymus gland;
- help reverse bone thinning in the aged by aiding in the absorption of calcium from the intestines;
- accelerate wound healing and tissue growth after burns, trauma, or surgery;
- reduce urea levels in the blood; and
- reduce free–radical formation by burning the extra fat that otherwise could become peroxidized in the body.

HGH has several jobs in the body. We try to bend its influence over fat–burning and muscle–building to our weight–loss advantage.

It's best to take it at night, since HGH release occurs within the first ninety minutes of sleep. During the night, while you are soundly sleeping, the HGH can safely burn off ounces of fat.

For the best results, these amino acids should be used in combination with a balanced, medium–calorie diet, daily exercise, and proper sleep.

Availability: Most health food stores and drugstores stock various combinations and individual amino acids.

They usually combine twice the amount of L–arginine as L–ornithine.

Dosage: L–arginine 500 mg and L–ornithine 250 mg. The instructions are usually on the bottle. Take one or two at night before bedtime.

Another formula combines the following: L–arginine 1200 mg, L–ornithine, 900 mg, L–lysine 1200 mg. Take one or two at bedtime.

While still another formula acts to combine the L–arginine and L–ornithine with vitamin B–3, vitamin B–6, and the amino acid L–tryptophan. Again, the directions are to take them at night.

The FDA does not recognize any of these formulas as diet aids.

Feel Full with Fiber

During World War II, the U. S. Army developed K–rations. They were to be used by the men in the field when kitchens could not be set up to offer hot meals. They were fairly nutritious and highly concentrated, but they had one very serious drawback. Although they were full of protein and other nutrients, they lacked the bulk needed to fill the stomach. Soldiers were dissatisfied and felt hungry after they had consumed all of their rations.

A new form of K–rations was then developed. This contained, in addition to the food, a quantity of methylcellulose. Methylcellulose is derived from the vegetable kingdom. It's a fiber that has the unique property of absorbing water. Soldiers were told to drink a glass of water with their K–rations. The water was absorbed by the methylcellulose, which then swelled in the stomach creating a feeling of fullness. This solved the problem of the "empty feeling," and the new K–rations were a success.

After the war, the use of methylcellulose and K–rations was forgotten until the idea of using the principle of water and fiber to create a full feeling was resurrected as a diet concept. Unfortunately, the public would not accept the idea of eating sawdust (what methylcellulose really was), even though the GIs had to.

The concept was and is a good one. Fiber provides bulk without calories and can perform other beneficial acts in the body. However, good as the concept is, it remained for science to come up with alternatives to sawdust!

The two best bets turned out to be natural materials. One, called glucomannan, derived from a plant root; the other, a microalgae called spirulina.

Glucomannan has been used in Japan for centuries, and spirulina has been a food source in Africa for at least that long. Both of them are very low in calories. Both are high in fiber. Both absorb water and create a feeling of fullness in the stomach. Both have a history of safety extending back thousands of years.

Both are available at health food stores or at drugstores at only a fraction of the cost of prescription diet pills.

This chapter will deal with glucomannan, spirulina, and the other fabulous food fibers that have a bearing on diet and health.

Once the stomach feels comfortably full, you can relax and go on with the pleasurable business of losing weight. You will be able to feel stuffed on 1200 calories a day!

Cellulose

There is certainly a public awareness of dietary fiber. Not a day goes by without some reference or advertisement or comment from nutritionists, medical scientists or food manufacturers about the benefits to be gained by including fiber as a good part of your diet.

But do you know as much about fiber as you should?

Man has learned that many plants are safe to eat and that the principal component of the walls of plant cells, which, linked together, make up the structural framework, is a substance called cellulose.

As I mentioned, it was a substance called methylcellulose which was used to fool the soldiers' stomachs during World War II.

By one definition, dietary fiber is the portion of the diet that does not contribute nourishment in any way as it passes through the gastrointestinal tract. Although it may not offer nutrients, it does contribute to general health in many ways. Dietary fiber is as important a diet–component as are proteins, fats, and vitamins. Dietary fibers include cereal and vegetable brans, pectin, lignin, gum, and purified cellulose.

While "cellulose" is a name that has been linked with trees and sawdust, perhaps unfairly, it does have an exact chemical definition. It is beta–1,4–glucan. It is a polysaccharide composed of carbon, hydrogen, and oxygen.

Many products, particularly in the pulp and paper industry, contain cellulose in varying proportions, but food products are restricted to the use of purified cellulose dietary fiber.

The advantage of cellulose as a dietary fiber, once it has been purified, is that it has fiber content of the highest amount. It is also tasteless and odorless.

Therefore, if a product contains methylcellulose as an aid to diet by virtue of its ability to absorb water and expand in the stomach, it is not to be avoided because its origin may have been wood pulp. Specifications have been written by the various regulatory agencies concerning the quality of the pulp.

Spirulina

An ancient nutrient, which may have been the first active microorganism on earth, may be one of the best weapons against obesity.

Blue–green microalgae have blossomed for millions of years, but only in the past few decades has technology been brought to bear on cultivating, harvesting, and distributing these plants as a broad–based food.

Only very recently has the weight–regulating ability of this food been un-derstood and applied to a diet program.

What Is this New Food Source Called?

It is called "spirulina" and it's a type of plankton.

What's Plankton?

Any free–floating microscopic plant organism or animal organism which drifts in the water currents is classified as plankton. In the ocean it is the beginning of the food chain. Spirulina is a blue–green aquatic vegetable–plankton found in alkaline waters in many different parts of the world.

Is There More than One Kind of Plankton?

There are thousands of species of algae, classified generally by size and color. There are blue–green, brown, red–brown, red, and so on. By size they are divided into macroalgae, and microalgae, by definition so small that they must be looked at with a microscope.

Spirulina has been singled out for attention because of its nutritive qualities and potential therapeutic uses.

Why Is This One Type So Special?

It is a direct link to the original photosynthetic food of the ocean where all life started. It is a rare mine of vitamins and minerals. It is 60–70 percent digestible protein. It is a natural source of vitamin B–12 from the vegetable kingdom, which is usually found only in food of animal origin. It is a recognized source of Beta–carotene, which the body converts into usable vitamin A. It contains the B–complex vitamins, plus substan-tial amounts of iron and other minerals. It is also a source of mucopolysaccharides, essential unsaturated fatty acids, nucleic acids, chlorophyll, plus some vitamin E.

The ancient Aztecs used spirulina as one of their staple foods. Their version, called "tecuilatl," was a mixture of the algae with maize or corn. In nature, the algae blooms periodically, as rainfall washes the necessary nutrients from the soil into the water.

A French botanist, Jean Leonard, working in the Sahara Desert in the early 1960s noticed the growth of the blue–green algae on Lake Chad. He associated it with blue–green "cakes" he had seen in native villages. On investigation he found that the natives had been mixing the algae with any available cereal grains (millet, corn) or with onions and spices to make slabs of food called "dihe." It appears that this practice had gone on for centuries.

How Is It Cultivated for Today's Uses?

Spirulina is a filamentous plant with single cells joined end to end, usually less than a millimeter long and a single cell wide. They are stacked end–to–end and take a spiral shape. That's why it's called spirulina.

It can be grown under cultivation on artificial closed–pond systems, dependent on the input of nutrients in solution and carbon dioxide. It will grow very rapidly under optimal conditions and can double its mass every few days. It can also be gathered from natural growing places, such as the Sahara, and Lake Texcoco in Mexico.

The July/August, 1980, issue of *Whole Life Times* reported that spirulina could double the amount of protein available to the world on a fraction of the world's land, while helping to restore a balanced environment to the planet.

Spirulina does not require the use of prime land to be cultivated. To get as much protein, twenty times the acreage planted with soybeans (the best vegetable crop) would be required. And it would have to be planted on the best available land!

All This Is Very Interesting But How Will It Help Me Lose Weight?

The drawback to most diets is the elimination of many necessary nutrients as you cut back on the amount of food your body is used to. The action you take causes Diet Panic, because vitamins, minerals, and trace elements, as well as desirable amino acids, are now in a shortened supply.

The system becomes drained with accompanying physical, emotional, and mental problems. Adding supplemental vitamins and minerals helps in most cases. However, there are those people who, for some reason or other, do not readily absorb or assimilate some nutritional substances. They will find that they still hunger for sweets or for salty foods, even after they have eaten a meal.

You're Talking about What Happens to Me on a diet!

You're not alone.

The diet victim ends up pacing the kitchen, in an endless search for foods or combinations of foods that will satisfy the messages coming from the hungry body.

Sometimes the use of L–phenylalanine or L–tyrosine can answer these needs by retraining the chemicals in the brain. However, we are all so individual that what will work splendidly for one person will not do a thing for someone else with a slightly different genetic background. Cravings for ice cream (sweet), or pickles (sour–acid), or peanut butter (salt), or bananas (sweet) are not uncommon.

What's the Answer?

Spirulina can be one answer to this problem.

Although many over–the–counter diet tablets contain drugs and chemicals that depress the appetite for a short period of time, the side effects can be dangerous and unpleasant. Also, the body quickly builds up a tolerance and the tablets lose their effectiveness in a few weeks.

Spirulina contains phenylalanine—the main ingredient of most over–the–counter reducing pills—in its natural vegetable form.

When you take it, it quickly works to release the appetite–killing chemicals within the brain and stomach. However, it has no dangerous side effects, as over–the–counter pills most definitely do. It is a low calorie supplement, a natural hunger–satisfier, and an aid to cleansing and fasting.

Availability: It is available in most health food stores and in some drugstores.

You can buy it in tablet form, as a powder, as a diet formula, energy food, pasta, and as flakes to sprinkle on other foods. It is also included in stress–reducing supplements offered for sale in some health food stores.

The protein in spirulina is much easier to digest than most other protein foods and, as a result, it is absorbed very quickly. This quick absorption helps signal the brain at once that it has received a full supply of needed nutrients. This quick absorption also helps to keep the blood sugar at normal levels. Why is this so vital? Because your brain ordinarily reacts to low blood sugar levels by setting off the hunger pangs you hate. So keeping your blood sugar normal is essential to losing weight painlessly.

Dosage: You can adjust the dosage to suit your own individual needs. Try taking three of the 500 mg tablets (or the equivalent in any other form) with a full glass of water one–half hour before meals.

If this is the right dosage for you, and it succeeds in reducing your hunger or keeping it away, try reducing the amount to two tablets or even one tablet before meals.

Will I Feel Tired When Using Spirulina?

Usually not, because it also is capable of supplying the type of fuel the body needs for energy. Especially if you are taking supplemental vitamins and minerals, the combination of algae and supplements should take up the slack when you drop your caloric intake to diet level.

Do not be turned off by the color or the odor of spirulina. It smells like the ocean, but its taste is so bland that you may want to add some spices to it. Use garlic, onions, mustard, or any other herb you enjoy.

Millions of pounds of this algae are eaten yearly in Japan, Taiwan, West Germany, Eastern Europe, the USSR, Egypt, and India. All agree that this algae should be utilized as a food resource. There is no evidence of any negative side effects or complications with the use of spirulina.

The FDA has permitted it to be imported into this country as a food supplement, but has not classified it for any other purpose.

Glucomannan

As researchers learn more about health problems that relate to obesity (high blood pressure, diabetes, and others), they are exploring various means to overcome chronic obesity.

Although they have come up with many concepts, such as placing a balloon in the stomach, wiring the jaws shut to prevent eating solid foods, shutting off part of the stomach, and other bizarre ideas that can be as dangerous or more dangerous than the obese condition itself, these research "solutions" have not been able to outdo nature's dietary gifts.

Supplementing your diet with glucomannan not only makes good scientific sense, it also has a history of safety that goes back over two thousand years.

Glucomannan is derived from the edible root of the konjac plant (amorphophallus konjac), which is in the same family as another edible root that we are very familiar with, the yam. The Japanese have long cultivated and reaped the benefits of this plant.

The uses of the konjac are recorded in an ancient Japanese medical book called *Honzokomoku*, which lists medicinal herbs that have been in use for over two millennia. The roots were considered so valuable that they have been dried and preserved in the Japanese imperial treasury as a valuable commodity.

Konjac has been part of the foods brought into this country by the Japanese community and is found in certain groceries and supermarkets. You may see some of the konjac products in the Oriental section of your local store. The name can be "Yam threads," "Shirataki" noodles, or a form of cake called "Konnyaku." The offbeat taste and texture has not created a following among Occidentals.

However, modern processing methods have removed these minor drawbacks, and glucomannan is now extracted from the root and prepared for western tastes and uses.

All Very Interesting, but Why Should I Learn about It?

Because this simple Oriental compound helps people lose weight!

Availability: In most health food stores it is available in powder, capsule, cake, tablet, cookie, and candy forms.

Dosage: Glucomannan expands fifty to sixty times in size when it reaches the stomach.
The idea is to take about 1,000 mg. Usually they come in 500 mg capsules or tablets, so take two of them with eight ounces of water one–half hour before a meal.

The glucomannan gently swells in the stomach, bringing a feeling of fullness. When the stomach feels full, it sends a signal to the hypothalamus (the appetite–control center). The hypothalamus then, in turn, sends a return signal to reduce hunger and appetite. Because of the feeling of fullness and the presence of supplemental nutrients provided by the vitamin tablets you take, Diet Panic and Diet Stress do not set in.

People who follow this simple diet technique eat less food during meals and feel satisfied much more quickly.

So, According to the Use of Glucomannan, I Will Be Able to Cut Calories without Feeling Deprived!

Yes, you will automatically be able to eat less, because your stomach will be full and happy. Be sure to take smaller portions since each of us has a built–in command to finish all of the food on the plate. It began when we were children, and is a very difficult command to ignore.

Weight Loss without Will Power?

There is another theory why glucomannan can help you to lose weight.

Since glucomannan is in the stomach before you eat, when the food arrives, it is surrounded by the swelling mass. This coating helps to speed the food through the digesting area, so less of the food is available for absorption. That means less time for the body to absorb fats and sugars, the food parts mainly responsible for extra pounds.

Few people have the will power to abandon the foods they have eaten since childhood and learned to love. Few people feel comfortable sticking to a severe reduced–calorie diet no matter how obese they are or how badly they want to lose weight. Fewer still want to endure the hunger that *has* to ensue from a restricted diet—particularly when there are so many food temptations all around, all day long.

People who want to lose weight *don't want to be hungry or give up eating the foods they love!* But everyone who's ever been on a diet knows that hunger and temptation are everywhere, and will power fades when confronted with heady aromas and tantalizing tastes.

The Diet Crutch

Glucomannan helps when will power weakens. It helps to put you back in control of your own appetite. It helps to reset your built–in appetite regulator. It has a place in every diet regimen, and can make the difference between success and failure in achieving your ideal weight, no matter what diet program you choose.

What about the Calories from Glucomannan Itself?

Glucomannan itself cannot be absorbed.

Although it is a natural blend of two common carbohydrates (glucose and mannose), the molecules are connected in such a manner that the body cannot break them down and accepts glucomannan as fiber, with all of the good things connected to fiber.

Glucomannan, besides its diet help, also helps correct constipation, especially diet constipation. It can also help in cases of food allergy by helping to remove toxic substances from the digestive tract before they can penetrate the abdominal wall and enter the blood stream. Glucomannan acts as a "scouring pad" for the intestine—cleaning out the gut, helping keep only friendly bacteria in place

Other Possible Benefits

The Japanese use glucomannan for a number of reasons. The weight–control capacity is just one of its uses. They also use it to help regulate blood sugar levels.

People with high blood sugar levels (hyperglycemia) or low blood sugar levels (hypoglycemia) can have radical mood swings. They are also troubled by muscle weakness, dizziness, and/or nervousness.

Glucomannan can slow the release of sugar into the blood after a meal and can relieve the stress on the organs involved in controlling blood sugar levels.

Other studies, in both the United States and Japan, have shown not only significant weight loss in tested subjects but also measurable decreases in cholesterol and triglyceride levels, substances associated with arteriosclerosis and increased risk of heart disease.

As I have said, glucomannan also acts to cleanse the system as it moves along the digestive tract—carrying with it toxic substances, cholesterol, triglycerides, and other unwanted material out of the body.

Again, How Can I Add Glucomannan to My Diet?

Take about 1,000 mg of glucomannan one–half hour before meals. Make sure you take at least eight ounces of water with it. Adequate amounts of liquid are necessary to make the process work for you. Too little water will act against the swelling action and deprive you of the full benefits of glucomannan.

Some people may have been told to restrict fiber in their diet. In that case you will have to choose one of the other substances in the book. The same restriction applies to people with digestive tract disorders. Check with your doctor if you have any doubts.

If you are currently taking any prescription drugs or medication, consult with your doctor before using glucomannan. The fiber can interfere with the absorption of a drug, just as it can interfere with absorption of sugar.

The same caution applies if you are pregnant. Since the growing baby requires adequate nutrition, glucomannan is not the best choice to maintain weight during pregnancy.

Any diet requires a careful check to be sure you are obtaining adequate amounts of nutrients. Since glucomannan will block some of the absorption of calories, it will also block some of the absorption of nutrients. Also, since it speeds the transit of the food through the stomach, it cuts down on the amount of nutrients the body can absorb in that shorter space of time. All this is a help to you as far as losing weight, but you have to be careful not to cut down on nutrition.

Therefore, it is suggested that you have one meal a day without the use of the glucomannan. Take your vitamins with this meal as well, to insure absorption of the supplemental nutrients.

Some people can feel a bit bloated when they begin to use glucomannan. If that happens, just cut the dose in half for two or three days to let your system adjust to it.

Glucomannan is offered for sale as a dietary supplement and has not been approved by the FDA for any other purpose.

Food Fiber

Hunger and the need to eat are normal body mechanisms controlled by our most primitive brain, which can supercede the more modern brain under crisis conditions.

The desire to eat is as strong an urge as your sex drive. Because you need to eat to stay alive, your empty stomach will nag at you with hunger pangs, rumbling, growling, and gas attacks.

Taming the Growling Beast of a Hungry Stomach

In order to stop this reminder that your stomach demands filling, you have to put something in it or you will be bullied into eating. Filling your stomach and achieving the quiet peace of satiety is the job of substances like glucomannan, spirulina, and our western counterpart, fiber!

Bran fiber, for one, is the tough outer coating of the cereal grain. While it and other cereal grain fibers do not possess glucomannan's amazing power to swell in the stomach, fiber does make you feel full and less hungry when taken before a meal in supplement form or as part of a meal.

Fiber has the ability to modify hunger. Fiber can cleanse the digestive tract of toxins.

Fiber is more than just roughage for the purpose of mechanically flushing the bowels, although this attribute is normal to a diet containing a useful amount of fiber. It does much more for the human body than that alone. Research is still exploring fiber's functions in the body and finding some surprises.

In the seventeenth century, obesity was the fashion. Paintings of the era depict women of very ample proportions, and for about two hundred years most women were relatively obese in order to be in fashion.

This trend toward fat was not really a conscious decision of the Baroque period, but a result of new food–processing techniques that attempted to remove food as far as possible from its origin. The most significant contribution to fat was the milling of flour to remove every last bit of chaff (fiber or roughage).

The flour produced by this new milling process contained far more calories to the ounce than the older, unrefined flour. And another health–protector was left on the refiner's floor.

Fiber added satisfying bulk without unnecessary calories. People consumed more of the new flour in order to achieve a full stomach adding many more calories and more weight.

Fiber Facts

Fiber is defined as the undigestible cell walls of plants. It has been called roughage, bulk, plant residue, plantix, and unavailable carbohydrates. The medical profession defines fiber as dietary components that increase fecal bulk, or those parts of plant materials which are resistant to digestion by secretions of the human gastrointestinal tract.

From a chemical standpoint, total dietary fiber is composed of cellulose, hemicellulose, pectins, gums, lignin, and mucilages. All of the fiber parts do not appear in all plants, and all of the different fiber parts have different physiological effects when alone or in combination.

Cellulose exists in large amounts in grasses, legumes, and other forage plants. Dietary celluloses are essentially unchanged during food preparation and cooking.

Hemicellulose is a group of polysaccharides, which differs from cellulose in that it may be hydrolyzed by dilute mineral acids, and is not readily digested by the starch–digesting enzyme released by the pancreas (amylase). Hemicellulose has some properties similar to the gums.

It holds water, is partly digestible, and is capable of binding trace minerals and bile salts.

Lignin is a noncarbohydrate fiber. It is insoluble. Cabbage contains 6 percent lignin, while apples contain about 25 percent.

Pectin is from a group of water–soluble polysaccharides. Apples are 15 percent pectin.

Plant Gums are a mixed group of complex polysaccharides, which are essentially nondigestible by man.

Dietary fiber has the capacity to hold water when its surface and interior tissues are saturated with water. *So, a great deal of the beneficial effect of fiber on your diet has to do with the amount of water you drink.* Food fiber, since it absorbs and retains water during its passage through the alimentary canal, will keep food moist as it traverses the stomach.

The moistness of the food promotes the movement along the intestinal tract.

The quicker the movement, the less chance for sugars and fats to be absorbed and to be deposited in fat cells! That's one of the ways in which fiber acts to control weight.

The undigested fiber increases the bulk of the stool and stimulates the rectal reflex to get rid of waste material. This prevents assimilation at the other end of the colon.

Thanks for the Lessons on Fiber. Now, How Do I Use What I Know to Lose Weight?

You can add fiber to your diet by eating more fiber foods and by using fiber supplements. Manufacturers have not overlooked the convenience factor of carry–about products that contain fiber. These easily fit into a pocket or purse and can help the dieter either cut down on food at regular mealtime or resist snacks between meals.

The American diet, with its preponderance of refined carbohydrates and saturated fats, has contributed to the high incidence of diabetes, coronary heart disease, and obesity. Our main manufacturing companies have been more concerned with improving the color and the palatability of the food we eat and less concerned with nutritional value.

Plant fiber used to be thrown away or saved for the use of livestock. Now that we know that plant fibers play an important role in digestion, absorption, and metabolism, as well as general health, we don't throw the fiber away—but that does not mean that we have increased the amount of fiber–containing foods we eat. Knowledge without the wisdom of utilizing the knowledge is akin to ignorance!

Despite broad agreement in the nutritional and medical communities on the value of fiber, there is a great deal of resistance among individuals to increase their intake. Perhaps it is the lack of palatability or the difficulty in chewing fiber products. Some manufacturers are now packaging fiber with other tasty foods, such as raisins, nuts, and bits of fruit. This should increase public acceptance of fiber on a daily basis.

However, other manufacturers have capitalized on the idea of convenience and put together chewable fiber tablets or wafers.

Fiber includes cellulose, hemicellulose, lignins, pectins, gums, mucilages, and storage polysaccharides. The majority of plant fibers (such as cellulose, hemicellulose, and lignin) are insoluble and play their part in the health of the body due to their insolubility.

Pectins, on the other hand, can be digested or fermented in the colon. They form gelatinous masses in the presence of water. Because of their binding and water–absorbing quality, they are widely used in the food industry in the production of ice cream, sauces, salad dressings, and pie fillings.

The subject of fiber and its uses is a complicated one, and the people who manufacture fiber wafers have to exercise judgement when they combine various fibers for the desired dietary affect.

For example, consider the effect of eating an apple compared to drinking some apple juice. It's the pectin in the whole apple that helps you to feel satisfied. The juice, which is devoid of pectin, can never give you the feeling of fullness that the whole apple can.

A good fiber wafer will combine fibers from an assortment of foods. Look for pectin and various fruit fibers on the label.

Availability: Fiber supplements are available in health food stores in a number of forms. There are fiber tablets, fiber wafers, fiber crackers, fiber candy bars, fiber soups, and so on.

Dosage: If you want to use the fiber tablets, wafers, or crackers, chew them very well and make sure that you drink at least eight ounces of water with them.

Two or more tablets, wafers, or crackers one–half hour before meals with water is the usual dose.

There may be a bit of stomach growling or distension if you are not used to having fiber in your system. If this happens, reduce the amount that you are taking for two or three days and then begin again.

If I Want to Use Foods for Fiber, How Much Should I Add?

Most nutritionists recommend at least 30 to 45 gm of assorted fiber a day. That's a difficult amount to ingest as you will see from reading the following list:

Breads and Cereals

Each serving has about 2 gm of fiber:

Whole wheat bread	1 slice
Cracked wheat bread	1 slice
Rye bread	1 slice
All–Bran	1 tbsp.
Shredded wheat	1/2 pillow
Oatmeal (dry)	1 1/3 cups

Fruit Foods

Each serving has about 2 gm of fiber:

Apple	1 small
Cherries	10 small
Banana	1 small
Orange	1 small
Peach	1 small
Pear	1/2 small
Plums	2 small
Strawberries	1/2 cup

Vegetables

Each serving has about 2 gm of fiber:

Carrots	1/3 cup
Celery	1 cup
Green beans	1/2 cup
Broccoli	1/2 cup
Brussels sprouts	4
Potato	2–inch size
Lettuce (raw)	2 cups
Tomato (raw)	1 medium

Because of the lack of knowledge about fiber, most people assume that they are getting a sufficient amount. As you can see from the amounts contained in various foods, 30 gm of fiber daily might be a bit of a problem, unless you decide to supplement the food intake.

When you buy a fiber supplement, try to make sure that it contains fiber from various sources. The label should tell you how much fiber is in each portion (whether tablet or cracker), and what kind of fiber is within.

A good fiber supplement will contain fiber from wheat, bran, corn, citrus, and so on.

Unless your doctor has put you on a fiberless diet because of some gastrointestinal problem, you should incorporate fiber foods into your diet to lower your sugar and fat intake, to help lower cholesterol and triglyceride levels, and to help eliminate waste material.

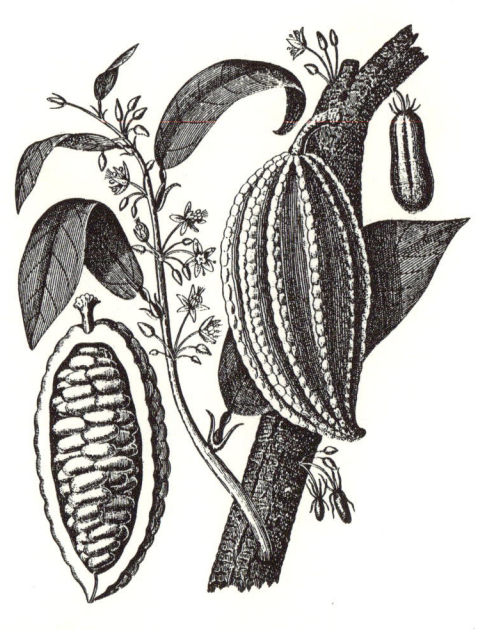

More Efficient Prostaglandins

Can you shed those pounds without pain and suffering, without starving yourself, without undue deprivation, without stretching your will power?

Gamma–Linolenic Acid (GLA)

Some say a new era is here, a new era of diet control, thanks to the natural magic of a substance called gamma–linolenic acid (GLA).

I repeat, if cutting back on calories is the answer to obesity, then why are so many people on low–calorie diets still overweight?

It's time to learn about GLA, one of the secrets of keeping Diet Panic out of your life while you shed your excess baggage.

It seems that GLA is a substance that calms Diet Panic. It restores you to your benevolent self and starts your body burning fat.

Scientists have long suspected that everybody has some kind of fat–burning mechanism, and now they have discovered that it comes in two parts. The first is the special kind of tissue called Brown Fat. It's called Brown Fat because it is brown in color. This makes it different from the fat the body burns, which is White Fat. The reason Brown Fat is brown is that it is loaded with large numbers of fat–burning motors, known as mitochondria. It is in these motors that White Fat is burned and that excess calories are consumed, instead of being stored away in fat cells. Under normal circumstances, when you eat, the brain tells your Brown Fat to burn off the extra calories.

But All People Are Not Equal When It Comes to Brown Fat!

Researchers have found ways to measure the activity of Brown Fat. They've discovered that thin people have active and well–functioning Brown Fat, but overweight people have Brown Fat with a low level of fat–burning activity.

This means that the Brown Fat in overweight people is not cooperating, not burning up the extra calories the way it should. And, since the calories aren't burned, the body has no choice but to store them away in the fat cells.

The other part of the fat–burning mechanism is a system called the "sodium pump." This system regulates the amount of sodium and potassium (essential minerals) that are in the body cells. They keep a balance between the two by pumping them in or out of the cells, depending on the concentration. Thousands upon thousands of enzymes take part in the operation of the pump and all of them require large amounts of energy to do their job.

The latest estimate is that between 25 and 50 percent of all available body energy is used to keep the pump running and in good condition.

What Has That To Do with My Diet?

The presumption is that if you are reading this book, you must have something to lose!

Thin people tend to have sodium pumps that work properly and efficiently, burning large numbers of calories. Overweight people have defective pumps that don't do their jobs very well and burn a lot fewer calories. *It is possible that many people, if not most, do not gain weight simply because they eat too much. Their bodies work against them, putting the pounds in storage instead of burning them.*

The important thing is *not* how many calories you take in but *how your body processes them.*

So, if you're counting on calorie reduction to do the trick, and your body has lost its ability to burn up the few calories you do eat, it will still store fat no matter how restricted the diet!

The only thing that your overweight, overstuffed body is crying out to you is this: "Help me. I need the raw materials that will assist me in burning up fat. Don't starve me—just fix the situation and I'll slim myself."

I Want To Help My Body! What'll I Do?

GLA is one of the natural aids you'll need, but it is hard to find in the foods you normally eat. It was first uncovered in mother's milk (admittedly not a regular part of any menu if you've over diaper age).

Mother's milk is the oldest and safest human food, and it is reasonable to assume that the GLA content plays a major role in the initial development of the infant. Cow's milk, on the other hand, contains very little GLA.

What Does This GLA Actually Do in the Body?

GLA is involved in the production of prostaglandins.

Prostaglandins are hormone–like substances that are manufactured in the body.

They are responsible for second–by–second control of almost ever body function.

They are the health controllers.

Prostaglandins cannot be stored, and every tissue manufactures them as needed. Their effect is split–second brief because they are inactivated by enzymes.

GLA is essential to good health and, in order to make it easy to understand, you'll have to compare it to the gasoline you put into your car.

If you put the best grade of gasoline into your tank, the car will run at peak efficiency.

If you put the poorest grade of gasoline in your car it will still run, but it will run badly. Coughing, spitting, burning oil, stopping and starting; eventually it will break down.

Your body must manufacture prostaglandins, but the quality of the prostaglandins depends on the raw materials supplied.

In the past, scientists used to think we all could make our own top–grade prostaglandins from an essential fatty acid (EFA) called linoleic acid. It is found in oils and fats. But, EFA is only the starting point. It's useless unless it is converted to other compounds by the body. Unfortunately, the types of fats we eat the most of block the formation of GLA.

We can make GLA out of linoleic acid, if that reaction is not blocked by trans–linoleic acid or by a shortage of vitamin B–6, zinc, magnesium, or insulin, or by certain genetic difficulties. It is not an easy process.

Although cis–linoleic acid is found in unprocessed vegetable oils and can be a source of GLA, commercial processing in standard American foods such as margarines, peanut butters, and hydrogenated fats (such as Crisco) creates the "trans" form, which blocks the utilization of GLA. This processing is done to keep the commercial products from "going bad" on the shelves, but doesn't help us in the prostaglandin production department.

Although this book is about weight loss, prostaglandins do much more for the body.

In the last few years, scientists have learned the functions of a number of them. The prostaglandin "E" and "F" families are the most important so far. The "I" family member, called PGI, is also of interest. One member of PHI–2, often called prostacyclin, is a cell regulator and anticlotting agent.

The numbers 1, 2, or 3 refer to the EFA used as the raw material for production. If GLA is used as a starting point, the number 1 indicates this.

The PG series that uses arachidonic acid (AA) (another fatty acid found in vegetable oils) is indicated by number 2.

The PG series made from eicosapentaenoic acid (EPA) (found in fatty fish and the subject of loads of research studies because it helps ward off coronary problems) is indicated by the number 3.

The prostaglandins made from GLA and EPA have desirable functions, often blocked by those made from arachidonic acid or linoleic acid.

PGE–1 and PGE–3 keep blood platelets from sticking.

PGE–2 promotes platelet aggregation or clumping, which may be the first step toward a clot.

A balanced diet should supply the appropriate fatty acids. However, many people consume too much AA and too little GLA and EPA.

This chapter is difficult to understand, so here's another look at the process.

Linoleic acid or arachidonic acid found in vegetable oils is first converted to gamma–linoleic acid, then to dihommo–linoleic acid and then finally to PGE–1.

The first step to gamma–linoleic acid is frequently blocked by trans fatty acids; by a lack of nutrients that normally help in the conversion; by a lack of enzyme delta–6–desaturase; by a lack of zinc, magnesium, vitamin B–6, biotin, or vitamin C.

Therefore, instead of beginning with linoleic acid, you had better begin the process with GLA found in evening primrose oil.

Oil of Evening Primrose

Scientists began to search for other sources of GLA. They knew that nature seldom puts all of its eggs into one basket, and what is found in one source is usually available somewhere else if you look hard enough. They looked, and found another source in the seeds of the evening primrose plant. Once they had found a source, they began to breed the plant to increase the GLA content.

"Down the Primrose Path" is an expression that is more apt here than when used to describe a flower–strewn future, dreamlike and unrealistic. But, when applied to the real evening primrose, is a good path to be on.

The evening primrose grows in dry fields from Labrador to Florida and west to the Pacific. It grows at sea level and up to an altitude of about nine thousand feet. It is a biennial, blooming from early summer to the first frost.

Its scientific name is Oenothera biennis, family Onagraceae. It is native to the United States, and the American Indians knew about it and its medicinal properties. They used it to treat skin diseases and inflammation, to drain bloating out of the body, to heal wounds, and to help those with asthma. The root was used as a sedative and a cough suppressant, it also was used as a pain killer and an astringent.

The Pilgrims soon discovered its medicinal use, and quickly transported seeds to England where it was known as a panacea. It was so venerated that it became known as the "King's Cure–All."

The seeds are very tiny and, in the beginning, had to be harvested by hand. They yield an oil that is about 9 percent GLA.

The most recent results of the use of evening primrose oil capsules come from the Department of Nutrition at the Tulane University School of Public Health in New Orleans, Louisiana.

Evening primrose oil was given for six weeks to twenty–three overweight individuals, one or both of whose parents was also obese.

Obesity was defined as a body weight at least 20 percent above the ideal for height and frame. Those with diabetes or other endocrine disorders were excluded.

The purpose of the test was to study whether evening primrose oil alone, without changes in the diet or exercise, would result in weight loss.

When the results were in, compared to a control group taking placebo capsules, those taking evening primrose oil capsules had demonstrated a significant weight loss even though calorie intake actually rose.

Skinfold thickness (a measurement of body fat) fell significantly at all three points tested. The percent of body fat lost calculated from the change in skinfold thickness was 2.4 percent.

Moreover, activity of the sodium pump increased in the group taking evening primrose oil, but not in the group taking the placebo capsule.

Availability: Evening primrose oil is usually available in 500 mg capsules at health food stores.

But, don't rush out and buy them! There's a better way to get GLA. Earlier I told you that evening primrose oil contains about 9 percent GLA. Now there's a product on the market that contains about 18 percent GLA. Many companies package it. Ask for GLA and read the label carefully. This, too, is available in your health food store.

Dosage: Follow the directions on the bottle.

Take six capsules daily (two with each meal). Check the label to make sure that each capsule contains at least 40 mg of GLA (240 mg daily).

Include a vitamin and mineral supplement that will supply at least: 1000 mg vitamin C; 25 mg zinc; 100 mg B-6; 50 mg B-2; 50 mg B-3 (niacinamide).

Cholesterol Control

Although cholesterol, in excess, is a problem to all people, it is a greater problem to the obese.

Cholesterol is a white waxy fat required for membrane structures in all animals and humans, and is the starting material for the synthesis of many important hormones in the body, including the sex hormones, cortisone, and others.

Cholesterol is so essential that the human body could not survive without it—which is probably the reason why every cell in the body can manufacture it.

Everyone is capable of producing all of the cholesterol needed by the body.

Vitamin D begins with cholesterol and so do the bile salts.

So Why Be Concerned about Dietary Cholesterol?

Because it is now established beyond any reasonable doubt that high blood cholesterol will increase your risk of having a heart attack and dying from coronary artery disease.

Equally well–documented is the fact that eating excessive cholesterol in the diet will raise the blood–cholesterol levels, and that eliminating cholesterol from the diet will reduce blood cholesterol.

Since coronary artery disease and heart attacks are directly related to blood–cholesterol levels, the more cholesterol you eat in your diet, the greater your chance of having a heart attack and dying.

Your chances of suffering from this disease are lessened by eating a diet that contains no cholesterol.

But, unless you are a strict vegetarian who eats no meat, dairy products, or eggs, it is virtually impossible to completely eliminate cholesterol from the diet.

Where, in the Diet, Does Cholesterol Come from?

Cholesterol is found in all dietary products that begin with animals. These include all meats and meat products, fish, seafoods, eggs, dairy products, lard, tallow, and all food products containing any or all of those ingredients.

Animal brains contain the highest percentage of cholesterol. The most commonly consumed next–highest sources are eggs and organ meats such as liver. All meats, whether fat or lean, including chicken, fish, turkey, and seafood, contain cholesterol in fairly high amounts. Also, cholesterol is found in all dairy products, especially those made from the fat portion of milk, such as butter, cheese, cream, and ice cream.

How Does It Threaten Life?

Mainly by contributing to atherosclerosis.

Atherosclerosis is primarily a disease of our large and medium–size arteries. It occurs when fatty deposits, called artheromatous plaques, appear in the inner layers of these vessels. These plaques are especially rich in cholesterol. As the disease progresses, the arterial walls become thicker, harder, and sometimes calcified. Obviously, these diseased arteries lose flexibility and sometimes can be easily ruptured. Also, the rough surface of the plaques can cause the formation of blood clots, known as thrombi. These thrombi can break away from their attachment to the vessel wall and become free–flowing clots known as emboli.

Emboli generally do not stop flowing until they come to a narrow point in the circulatory system. This plugging of smaller arteries impedes or prevents the life–sustaining flow of blood.

Atherosclerosis is the underlying disorder in most coronary heart disease and, in addition, plays a major role in cardiovascular disease (stroke).

During a ten year period ending in 1984, the National Heart, Lung and Blood Institute (NHLBI) studied what relationship, if any, existed between cholesterol and heart disease. The results of this investigation, involving over 3,800 male subjects, are quite revealing.

A principal finding of this study showed that the risk of heart attack deaths dropped 2 percent for every 1 percent reduction in serum cholesterol.

It is clear that cholesterol absorption is proportional to cholesterol ingestion.

But I Can't Become a Vegetarian, So What Can I Do?

Most of us can't become vegetarians. The principal food items that contain relatively high amounts of cholesterol are important sources of other nutrients, and they taste good! Most of us are reluctant to remove or drastically reduce these foods from our diet. And, consider the impact on Diet Panic and Diet Stress.

So, we turn to nature once again and find that nature has provided us with a sensible and easy way to reduce the absorption of the cholesterol component in these good–tasting foods.

What Are These Helpers?

They're called *phytosterols.*

They are natural cousins to cholesterol that are found in the plant kingdom, mostly in grains, nuts, seeds, and fruit. Among the various types of phytosterols that exist, three have been found to be of the greatest nutritional importance. They are called: beta–sitosterol, stigmasterol, and campesterol.

This is their natural distribution in common oils:

Vegetable oil	Beta–sitosterol	Stigmasterol	Campesterol
Corn	66%	6%	23%
Wheat	67	n.a.	22
Peanut	64	9	15
Sunflower	60	8	8

The difficulty in using these oils as a source of the phytosterols is that they are usually destroyed in processing. If you want to add more natural vegetable sterols to your diet you will need to use unrefined oils. However, they are also rich in calories. If you use them, make sure to increase your intake of antioxidants such as vitamins A, C, E, beta–carotene, zinc, selenium, and other nutrients.

You can avoid the extra calories and the inconvenience of added purchases by getting a concentrate of natural sterols in tablet form.

Before I Go Out and Buy These Tablets, What Exactly Do They Do?

The majority of the scientific evidence gathered from animal and human studies suggests that phytosterols consistently delay and reduce the absorption of dietary cholesterol into the circulation.

So far, in spite of several investigations, the exact blocking mechanism is unclear—except that it works!

It may be due to formation of a non–absorbable cholesterol–phytosterol complex in the intestine; reduction in the solubility of cholesterol; inhibition of cholesterol uptake at the site of absorption in the intestine.

In other words, when phytosterols and cholesterols are combined during a meal, a certain percentage of the cholesterol will be blocked from the blood stream and forced to leave the body along with the waste material.

Availability: These tablets can be found in health food stores and drugstores.

Dosage: A daily intake of at least 300 mg (based on the beta–sitosterol content of the tablets) taken with meals (because it must be present along with the cholesterol) can have a significant effect on serum cholesterol.

But, you can't rely on the tablets alone!

They'll help, but you have to do a little cutting back on cholesterol–laden foods along with it. That means more vegetables, fruits, and nuts; less meat and dairy products. Not to the point where it irritates you, but definitely a reduction from your previous dietary amounts.

Other cholesterol fighters that should be included in your diet include: fiber, fish and fish oils, garlic and onions, avocado oil, and, of course, a good exercise program.

The FDA has not commented on the ability of phytosterols to lower serum cholesterol.

Glucose Tolerance Factor, Insulin, and Body Fat

The role of glucose tolerance factor (GTF) in body fat appears to indicate that anyone having a weight problem should concentrate on reducing with the aid of high quality foods rich in GTF, and should use GTF in supplement form.

GTF is a vital compound that helps control blood sugar. This new supplement can be good news for millions of people who have a craving for sweets.

In 1955, W. Mertz and K. Schwartz found that feeding small amounts of brewer's yeast to glucose–intolerant rats resulted in making those rats normally glucose tolerant. Therefore, it was concluded that the brewer's yeast contained a special ingredient that could improve the condition of laboratory animals suffering from abnormal sugar metabolism. This unknown ingredient was called GTF.

Later research identified chromium as one of the major components of GTF.

Chromium? That's the Shiny Stuff on Car Bumpers

That's right, chromium is part of the metal alloy that protects metal from rust. It's also used in industrial dyes. But, in the human body, chromium has the critical role of working with insulin to allow body cells their regular flow of glucose.

Chromium is crucial, irreplaceable, and often overlooked as an essential nutrient.

Scientists have discovered that there is a widespread chromium deficiency in the United States. The symptoms can begin as anxiety and low energy levels, and extend all the way to uncontrolled diabetes at the extreme.

The body's preferential energy source is glucose. All of the cells in the body need energy. All of the cells function very poorly on any other source of energy (except the brain cells, which can use glucose *and* glutamic acid).

Yet, for glucose to enter most body cells, the conditions must be just right for the glucose to pass through the cell membrane. Insulin, cyclic adenosine monophosphate (AMP), a special hormone, and GTF must be present at the right time and in the right quantities to facilitate the cell–wall penetration.

If no glucose enters the cell, the cell—requiring energy to live—begins to burn protein and fat.

Although the idea of trying to burn protein and fat might seem to be a good idea to someone interested in losing weight, *in this case it's destructive.*

The use of protein for energy causes tissue–wasting. Energy levels are low and erratic. There is poor circulation in the kidneys and the extremities, resulting in kidney failure or gangrene, as the body literally eats itself.

When the cells burn fat for energy as a replacement for natural glucose, excess fats in the bloodstream make the body a prime candidate for blocked arteries and heart disease.

All of this can come from an inability to properly utilize glucose as the primary fuel for energy.

Of all the trace minerals we need for good health (zinc, calcium, potassium, selenium, and so on), only chromium gradually disappears as we mature. We are born with a high concentration of this essential mineral, with minute amounts in our tissues and in the blood. The chromium forms a partnership with nicotinic acid (vitamin B–3 or niacin), the amino acids of glutathione (glutamic acid, glycine, and cysteine) and itself in its trivalent form.

GTF can be absorbed directly from food. Foods such as brewer's yeast (the richest source), mushrooms, wheat germ, oysters, certain cheeses, whole wheat bread, liver, corn oil, beets, fresh fruit, and chicken breasts contain small amounts, but only about 1 percent of dietary chromium is absorbed. The efficiency of conversion in usable form varies from person to person.

A deficiency can arise either because GTF is not in the food you eat, or you can't put the pieces together efficiently. The aging process also causes a significant decrease in GTF in many people.

GTF chromium is removed when food is refined. It is unfortunate that the further we remove food from the way nature meant it to be, the more problems we create for ourselves.

During experiments to discover the structure of GTF, it was learned that GTF significantly decreased cholesterol and triglycerides in diabetic and chromium–deficient animals. H. A. Newman and others verified that GTF may then be important in removing arterial plaques in man. (*Clinical Chemistry*, 24 [1978]:541.)

The reversal of cholesterol deposits is accomplished by lowering the blood cholesterol and increasing high density lipoprotein (HDL)—the cholesterol carrier that scavenges cholesterol and carries it back to the liver for disposal.

There are two cholesterol ferries in the body. One, called low density lipoprotein (LDL), delivers cholesterol around the body and the other, HDL, removes it from the body. The higher the ratio of HDL to LDL, the less chance of heart trouble.

Said one writer: The more garbage trucks (HDL) you have than delivery trucks (LDL, the better condition your arteries will be in and the fewer problems you'll have with plaque.

Tests cited in the *American Journal of Clinical Nutrition*, November 1980, link chromium deficiency with atherosclerosis, coronary heart disease, obesity, and hypoglycemia.

According to M. L. Newbold, M. D. chromium is useful in preventing and lowering blood pressure. It also helps prevent hardening of the arteries. This means that chromium helps fight the mental changes accompanying senility (*Meganutrients and Your Nerves*. New York: Berkeley Books, 1981).

Availability: You can get tablets of GTF at your health food store or drugstore.

Dosage: Normal maintenance levels run about 500 mcg a day.

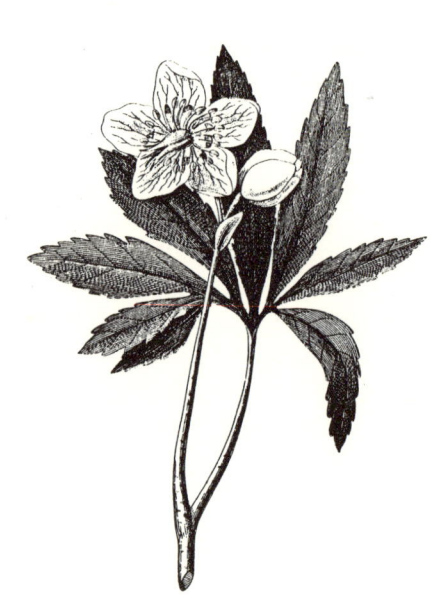

Help from the Land and from the Sea

Seaweeds include many useful species that may be eaten directly, or from which certain elements may be removed for nutritional purposes.

Like land plants, seaweeds (better called "sea vegetables") contain photosynthetic pigments, and develop my means of photosynthesis from the sun's energy. But, since they do not have the differentiation into roots, stems, and leaves, as land plants do, sea vegetables utilize energy more efficiently.

Kelp

We are most familiar with kelp. It is a remarkable food containing more mineral matter and vitamins than many well–advertised proprietary health foods, with the added advantage of being grown in the sea without the addition of artificial fertilizers.

Kelp acts on obesity mainly through the thyroid gland, which it tends to normalize. Thyroid gland malfunction, even on a small scale, can contribute to obesity on one hand or to extreme thinness on the other hand. Hence, a normal thyroid helps to maintain normal weight.

One function of the thyroid is to replenish energy, which is accomplished in cooperation with other endocrine glands.

It has been determined that there is a definite connection between our energy and our intake of iodine. In kelp we have a perfectly natural source of all the iodine we need.

If you think there is no connection between dieting and energy, think again. More people have been hurt by energy loss and body damage due to unwise caloric intake than have been helped by dieting. That is the reason I have devoted so much space to energy replenishment along with dietary nutrients. You cannot starve the body without doing some damage unless you take steps to provide *all* of the nutrients needed, from some source other than food, and restore the balance to all of the organs, tissues, and body systems.

Not only does kelp help heal a problem thyroid, but it also has a healing and normalizing effect on the nervous system, arteries, colon, liver, gall bladder, and fat cells.

Kelp can also exert a calming effect on the mind and body by relieving nervous tension. When nervous tension is marked, there is excitability and irritation. Sleeping becomes a problem, draining vitality.

In addition to iodine, kelp contains calcium, phosphorus, iron, sodium, potassium, magnesium, sulphur, chlorine, copper, zinc, and manganese, plus traces of rare minerals.

By increasing the body's metabolic rate, iodine causes an increase in physical and mental energy.

Quite recently it was reported that some of the ingredients in kelp can help to detoxify heavy metals, such as cadmium, lead, and mercury, which are poisonous to the body.

Availability: Kelp is available in tablets and granules at health food stores and in drugstores. (Comment: if you suspect that your weight problem is due to an underactive thyroid gland you must check first with your doctor. He may prescribe tablets containing thyroid or a synthetic compound that acts to stimulate thyroid function.)

Dosage: Follow manufacturer's directions.

The Seaweed Diet

The most common forms of seaweed are dulse and kelp. Although most seaweed available in health food stores come from Japan, the seaweed harvest off the American coast will do just as well.

Seaweed is unusually high in protein, and contains all forty–three trace minerals.

It also contains sodium alginate, which is a buffer against almost any harmful substance you can imagine: from pollution, smog, carbon monoxide fumes to even nuclear radiation.

Potassium is another valuable constituent. It initiates the healing process in the kidneys and the heart.

Seaweed boosts the function of the thyroid gland, which regulates weight. Seaweed speeds up metabolism to help regulate weight and also influences the parathyroid gland to better absorb the calcium the seaweed provides. So the extra benefit is to get stronger bones and teeth.

Availability: Seaweed is found in many health food stores.

Dosage: It can be cooked like spinach or added to soups. Use seaweed as you would a leafy green vegetable, in amounts to suit your taste.

Chlorella

There is a small, one-celled algae called chlorella that is a power-house of proteins, vitamins, and minerals. It gets its name from *chlor* for green and *ella* for small. It contains more chlorophyll than any other edible plant, and contains 60 percent good-quality protein.

Frequently, dieters are in need of a detoxification process, some way to get rid of accumulated waste material. Chlorophyll is well known for its detoxification abilities. The first comprehensive report on the ther-apeutic uses of chlorophyll was published in the *American Journal of Surgery* in 1940. This study reported on chlorophyll's use in fighting skin problems.

A person doesn't have to wait long after taking chlorella to discover its detoxification properties. Within a few days the bowels begin to func-tion much better than before.

***Availability*:** Chlorella is stocked in health food stores and drug-stores.

Dosage: Use according to manufacturer's instructions.

Chlorella is rich in nutrients and protein. It is useful as part of a weight-loss program. When used as such it should be taken with at least eight ounces of water. Meals should consist, for the most part, of vegeta-bles, cereals, salads, and fruits.

Note: Also see the Epilogue.

Wheat Grass

This grass is high in fiber and protein. It contains chlorophyll and other nutrients characteristic of deep green, leafy vegetables. Most people in societies like ours eat little or no green leafy vegetables, and those who do don't eat anywhere as much of them as did our ancestors.

We should supplement our diets with green roughage foods like con-centrated, dehydrated wheat grass, or barley. The young wheat plant is harvested when it is about eight inches tall and is more like a green grass than the golden wheat we picture in our minds.

The prophet Isaiah declared more than three thousand years ago that "all flesh is grass." Wheat grass, because it is actually the reservoir of nutrients for the growing embryo of grain, is among the richest of all grasses. Since it is harvested at an early age, wheat grass is more similar to a highly concentrated leafy vegetable than to the grain it was to become.

Besides being a concentrated source of the nutrients associated with green leafy vegetables, wheat grass is high in fiber. When taken before meals with a large glass of water, it expands at least fifteen times its original volume in the stomach to help you feel full. This enables you to control your appetite and consume less food at each meal.

Availability: Found in health food stores.

Dosage: Wheat grass tablets do not contain sugar. Use four to ten tablets with each meal with a full glass of water. You can start by taking two tablets and gradually build up to a maximum of ten. Or, follow manufacturer's instructions.

Barley

Young barley leaves contain a juice that is a pleasant source of vitamins, minerals, and enzymes. According to an analysis made by the Resource Association Office of Science and Technology, and Japan Food Analysis Center, the juice contains thirty times as much vitamin B–1 as does milk, over three times as much vitamin C and six times as much carotene as does spinach. It has eleven times as much calcium as cow's milk, nearly five times the iron found in spinach, seven times the vitamin C in oranges, plus 80 mcg of vitamin B–12.

The juice is also a rich source of chlorophyll and an assortment of other vitamins and minerals.

Several million Japanese are taking it. They have been mixing barley juice powder with water, juice, milk, or some other beverage. Its enzymes help digestion and loosening of hard fat. Its daily use helps solve a number of problems associated with obesity.

Availability: Barley can be found in health food stores in juice form, and in tablets or granules.

Dosage: Follow manufacturer's instructions.

Chlorella, wheat grass, or barley juice do not affect the thyroid gland the way that kelp does; therefore, they do not directly influence metabolism. They do help restore normal bowel movements during a dietary procedure, and do help provide nutritional support.

Chlorella and wheat grass may be used to cut appetite when taken before meals with sufficient water. Barley juice is restorative to a system that needs to get the most nutrients with the least amount of digestive effort.

It will take trial and error to discover which is best–suited for you.

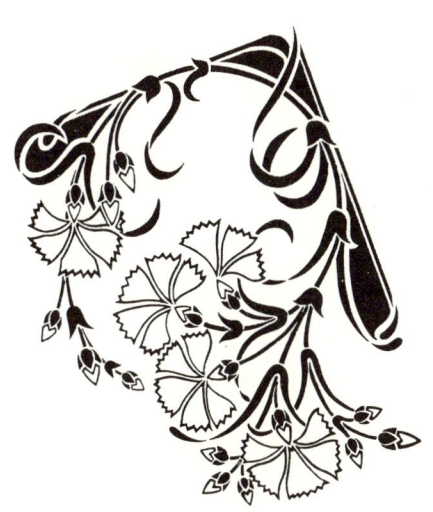

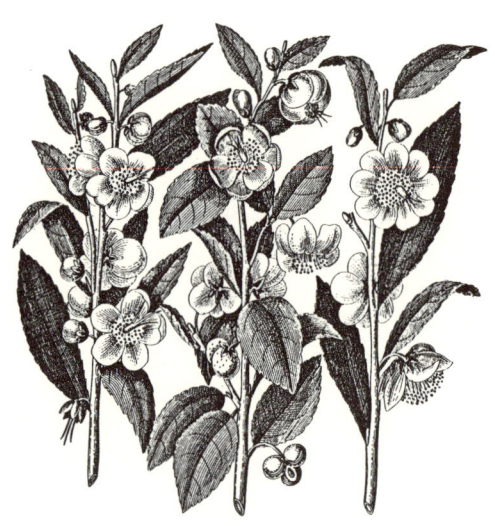

Combined Nutrient Formulas and Other Aids

Many combinations of nutrients are available on the market, and most of them have some good points to offer to the dieter. Usually they are combinations of well–known substances, with a history of help to dieters based on folk tales.

Nutrient Formulas

One formula combines papaya, garlic, and kelp. Natural foods can alter the body chemistry. Papaya contains a substance called papain. Papain is capable of splitting protein, is considered to be an aid to digestion, and will affect the caloric measure of ingested food.

Garlic has been said to have an amazing number of benefits. One such is the ability to clear the bloodstream of collected fats. This fat–clearing process contributes to weight loss, in that fats will be carried away in your body's waste products and not stored in the cells.

Kelp is a natural source of iodine. The iodine is needed by the thyroid gland, which governs the basic metabolic rate (the speed at which food is burned for energy). If there is a problem with the thyroid gland resulting in some slowdown in the basal metabolism rate, it is possible that kelp will be able to provide one answer.

This formula of natural substances, when combined with a limited diet and an increase in exercise, can be of help to many people who want to lose a few pounds, but not necessarily for those who are more than 15 percent over their best weight.

Another combination of natural substances designed to keep your energy level up while the pounds go down utilizes bee pollen, octacosonal, spirulina, and ginseng.

These four substances can give you energy without resorting to the use of artificial stimulants. Each has a history dating back thousands of years. Although the combination may be new, the individual substances have been used in home medicines with an admirable safety record.

Bee pollen is one of the most effective energy foods known. It is a complete food, containing sixteen vitamins, sixteen minerals, eighteen enzymes, eighteen amino acids, and twenty–eight trace elements. All of the nutrients are balanced. It is a rich source of protein and energy.

Octacosanol is an important energy–releasing food substance derived primarily from wheat. For those exhibiting an allergy to wheat–derived substances, there is octacosanol that has been derived from spinach. This is just as good as the wheat product. Octacosanol has been shown to improve strength, endurance, glycogen storage, and the ability to utilize oxygen more efficiently.

Spirulina is a tiny freshwater plant (vegetable plankton) that may be nature's most perfect source of complete protein, containing all of the essential amino acids. It also contains vitamins A, E, and B–complex; minerals; enzymes; chlorophyll; and vital trace elements. It is a prime source of vitamin B–12.

Ginseng is the famous herb that has been used for thousands of years to enhance both physical and mental energy levels and to increase endurance.

Nutrient combinations and theories abound.

Still another formula combines the following: potassium chloride, L–tyrosine, glucomannan, grapefruit, and octacosanol.

The enzymatic action of grapefruit on the body appears to start a fat–burning process that is boosted by the amino acid L–tyrosine (found in meat and cheese). This is said to be due to the conversion of L–tyrosine into the neurotransmitter norepinephrine, an appetite–inhibiting brain chemical.

Glucomannan further suppresses appetite by virtue of its ability to expand in the stomach (provided a sufficient amount of water is taken with this formula), producing a feeling of fullness. Glucomannan also provides fiber to support more efficient emptying of the bowels.

Potassium chloride is added to control excess fluids in the body and to also support the working of the adrenals.

Octacosanol, the ergogenic factor derived from wheat germ, is present to help put back the energy that dieters usually lose when the amount of food intake is restricted.

Some formulas also utilize psyllium (a natural laxative) and kelp (as a source of natural iodine to stimulate the thyroid gland).

Some weight loss products utilize a substance called guar gum. Guar gum is a fiber product extracted from the seeds of the Cyamopsis tetragonolobus found in India and Pakistan.

It is a natural dietary fiber in the form of indigestible carbohydrate that can absorb up to sixty times its weight in water.

Because it is not digestible, guar gum increases the bulk of matter in the stomach (provided enough water is taken with it). It remains in the stomach for a period of time, imparting a feeling of fullness that will help to discourage snacking between meals.

It then passed into the small intestine, which can absorb fats, calories, and carbohydrates. At the same time, studies show that guar gum acts to prevent sudden increases in the level of blood glucose and the secretion of insulin, which occur when food is passes too quickly through the body. It also can help to reduce elevated serum cholesterol, another plus to obese individuals.

As it continues into the large intestine, it can absorb harmful substances. The expanded bulk of the guar gum speeds the matter through the intestine, reducing the time that the fecal matter is in contact with the intestinal membrane, and thus normalizes bowel function.

Availability: Guar gum is available separately in tablet or packet form or as part of a reducing formula with other substances. It can be found in health food stores and drugstores.

Dosage: Use as directed by the manufacturer.

Some variations use grapefruit. It is said that there are substances contained in grapefruit which stimulate enzyme activity and help the body digest and eliminate fat.

However, it is not convenient to eat a grapefruit at every meal or to carry one around with you for lunch. So, some companies have used concentrated grapefruit extract plus other nutrients.

These formulas are basically the same, but with some variations of the synergistic nutrients that accompany it, such as apple cider, vinegar, kelp, lecithin, or vitamin B–6.

The apple cider, vinegar, and lecithin work with the grapefruit extract to break down fat and cholesterol in the body. Kelp provides iodine, a mineral essential for the thyroid gland. The combination of these four ingredients act as a gentle diuretic to help rid the body of excess water.

The next formula adds some amino acids: grapefruit, glucomannan, kelp, lecithin, apple cider vinegar, vitamin B–6, L–tyrosine, and L–phenylalanine. They are in such a pure form that within thirty minutes they not only reduce hunger pangs, but also produce a hormone that "convinces" your brain that you've already eaten enough.

Availability: Found in health food stores and drugstores.

Dosage: Follow instructions on package label.

The next formula has double fiber: grapefruit concentrate, glucomannan, guar gum, vitamin C, L–phenylalanine, and L–tyrosine.

Availability: Try health food stores and drugstores.

Dosage: Read labels and read directions carefully when you buy any reducing formula. Remember! If the label shows any type of fiber you must have a sufficient amount of water to activate it. Drink at least eight ounces of water, and perhaps a bit more each time you take a dose. Follow manufacturer's instructions.

The Garcinia Cambogia Fruit

The search for a good method of dieting that doesn't put too much strain on will power is not restricted to the United States.

The people of Southeast Asia, at least those who emulate the Western world, regard obesity as a problem. Their researchers have investigated the local flora and have come up with an interesting substance that is extracted from the rind of an edible fruit known as Garcinia cambogia (called the Brindall berry in the United States).

The tree is a relative of our native evergreen, but looks like a fruit tree. The berry contains natural fruit and fibers, and the locals use the dried rind as a flavoring or condiment.

The rind is also a source of a substance called hydroxycitric acid, and it is this substance that appears to be an effective adjunct to any weight loss program.

How Does It Work?

Theoretically, the hydroxycitric acid moderates the appetite by acting on peripheral gastrointestinal sites. It appears to lower fatty acid synthesis, resulting in lower body fat levels.

How Effective Is It for Weight Loss?

Over a half–dozen clinical studies have been conducted in laboratories. The results show reductions of up to 45 percent in food intake when the Brindall berry was given orally.

Is It Safe?

The berry has been eaten for years in Asia without any harmful effect, and there have been toxicity studies down as well, which prove its harmless character.

It Sounds Great but This Is Not Just Another Vegetable Laxative Is It?

Most diets do contain stimulants or laxatives, but this is just a pleasant tasting purple fruit rind extract without stimulant or laxative components.

Hydroxycitric acid is effective in reducing appetite and weight gain without having to resort to either stimulants or laxatives.

Also, when Brindall berry is used for dieting there is no "rebound" effect when it is discontinued. You never want to go on an eating binge.

And, it has been observed that hydroxycitric acid, because it inhibits fatty acid production, also reduces serum cholesterol and triglyceride levels up to 30 percent.

Availability: This is one product you may have to look for. Not all health food stores know about it and not all of them have it in stock. If you ask around, you will be able to find it.

Dosage: Take one or two tablets before meals with a glass of water. Give the Brindall berry formula a chance to dissolve in the stomach before you sit down to eat.

The FDA has registered this product as a dietary supplement and not as an aid to reducing.

What follows is a more complete story on: bee pollen, octacosanol, fructose, alpha–ketoglutarate, and vitamin B–15.

These substances are found in many reducing formulas. They also may be used in conjunction with any reducing program you may choose. When putting together your own formula you can add more or less of any ingredient, depending on your personal need.

Bee Pollen

This supplement can be found in two forms. One is produced by virtue of the hard work of the bee as it gathers pollen and brings it back to the hive. The other is from the hand of man, who visits the flowers before the bee gets to them and takes the pollen.

First, we will discuss pollen gathered by the bee.

A human being has to labor many hours to collect a thimbleful of the ultrafine powder, but a hive of bees can gather over sixty pounds or more each spring. These team workers extract pollen by visiting flowers and collecting the powder on their body. The delicate particles cling to the surface. Grains of pollen taken from the flower are mixed with a bit of nectar, formed into a tiny ball, tucked into a special sac and carried back to the hive to serve as food for developing larvae.

For many centuries pollen has been esteemed as a valuable nutrient in many corners of the world. It has been called both a food and a medicine. Athletes of ancient Greece and Rome ate great quantities of it to increase stamina and prolong the years of youthful vigor.

It also has its place in mythology as the magical food responsible for the immortality of the gods. It has their daily food, called ambrosia, a savory blend of honey and beebread (pollen).

Devotees have voiced grandiose claims for bee pollen, calling it a youth promoter and an energizer for use during dieting, when the reduction of calories calls for nutrient–dense foodstuffs.

("Nutrient–dense" refers to the relationship of nutrients to calories. Bee pollen is nutrient–dense. It gives the best ratio of nutrition to calories. Exactly the opposite of "junk foods.")

According to information recently received, Russia, Poland, Hungary, and Yugoslavia are investigating the use of bee pollen on a scientific basis. This really is no new thing since it was in the 1940s that Dr. Nicolai Tsitsin, biologist and botanist, conducted longevity tests in the Soviet Union. A region in the Caucasus was the center of long life, with a large number of people reaching the age of one hundred and older. Tsitsin wrote to a large number of centenarians, asking them to disclose their age, occupation, and principal food. When the returns were tallied, an unusually large number of them reported that they were beekeepers by trade, and all of them listed honey as their main food.

Then Why Not Write about Honey Instead of Pollen?

Because Tsitsin was not satisfied with that explanation. He knew of many people in other parts of Russia who bought honey and used it regularly without living as long as the beekeepers did. Something else had to be happening.

Further investigation showed his suspicions to be correct. For economic reasons the beekeepers had to sell the pure honey they gathered from their hives. After all, it was their main source of income. What they kept for themselves and ate daily was the waste matter that collected on the bottom.

This waste matter was mostly pollen that had fallen from the bee as it entered the hive, plus a small quantity of honey! It was this factor Dr. Tsitsin held responsible for the power of longer life.

In 1976, a document was prepared by the Department of Physiology at the Far East Institute of the Soviet Academy of Science. Entitled "Bees in the Service of Humanity," by Dr. Naum Petrovitsch Joirisch, this paper extolled the virtues of pollen. The author called it a treasure–house of nutrition and regenerative power. He described it as a perfectly–balanced food containing all twenty–two amino acids, twenty–seven mineral salts, a full range of known and unknown vitamins, and a collection of the most needed enzymes.

The document goes on to examine bee pollen's specific therapeutic values for human beings. In a description perhaps a bit too poetic, but nonetheless accurate, Dr. Joirisch calls pollen..."this marriage of blossom and bee (which) contains highly prophylactic and therapeutic properties." Bee pollen is a strong biological stimulant. It has regenerative properties for the organism. Its use in experiments with aging people seems to help restore morale, a sense of spiritual well-being, and actual physical health. It firms aging and lifeless skin. Among all age groups many of the ailments that responded favorably to bee pollen were chronic colitis, high blood pressure, and allergies. What this study revealed is part of the reason bee pollen is used so often as a dietary adjunct.

According to further studies conducted in the Soviet Union, each adult bee brings about four million grains of pollen back to the hives each hour via pollen baskets on the rear legs. Once the pollen is unloaded, young bees pour honey on it to protect it from the air. The queen will lay eggs as long as there is a supply of honey–coated pollen. If the supply is cut off for any reason, the queen will stop her egg–laying until a sufficient supply has been stored.

Other countries have also studied pollen. Dr. Emil Chauvin of the Institute for Bee Culture in Burres–sur–Yvette, France, tested mice on a diet exclusively of bee pollen. The animals showed no ill effects and demonstrated greater energy and an increased rate of reproduction.

When pollen was given to children and adults, it proved to be extremely beneficial in a number of serious conditions, including constipation, diarrhea, colic, and anemia. It also hastened convalescence.

Athletes, other than Russians, have also used pollen to help their efforts. Olympic Gold Medal sprinter Steve Riddick; Finland's Lasse Viren, winner of both the 5,000– and 10,000–meter races at Montreal; and our own Mohammed Ali.

Now we will examine the use of pollen gathered by man.

Why not use bee–gathered pollen?

It is agreed that pollen is one of the most important substances given to us by nature. It is also agreed that pollen is a valuable food supplement.

However, some people think that pollen collected by bees may be contaminated with pollutants that can cause allergic reactions among individuals sensitive to a particular flower.

So, machinery has been designed to take the pollen from the flower before the bee can get to it.

Like cutting out the middle man!

Availability: Bee pollen pellets are found in health food stores and drugstores.

Dosage: This is one answer I cannot give. Pollen is expensive and small amounts are included in many balanced diet formulas. If you want to buy pollen pellets and use them with meals as an extra nutritional source, it depends a lot on your pocketbook. Follow package instructions.

Octacosanol

By definition, octacosanol is an osolated, biologically active factor of wheat germ oil. It is a natural substance that improves endurance, speeds up reaction time, provides glycogen to muscles and strengthens them. It is considered to be an ergogenic (energy–releasing substance).

Octacosanol may increase fertility and prevent spontaneous abortion, lower cholesterol, and aid in the treatment of neurological disorders.

It also appears to be extremely helpful in weight reduction, through its ability to relax the nerves of your stomach. Otherwise, when your stomach loses it habitual fullness, these nerves tense up and drive you crazy with hunger pains. Octacosanol also increases the metabolic rate and reduces muscle tension.

If It's in Wheat, then Why Do I Have to Buy a Supplement?

Most of the food we consume in America has been processed to the extent that there is a complete or partial removal of up to twenty–five different nutrients.

Then the producing company puts back five or six nutrients and tells the public that the product is "enriched."

One such vital factor that is removed during the making of white flour is the substance known as octacosanol. But, even if processing didn't take it out of our food, we couldn't get the amount that is concentrated into supplement form. It would take over 4.5 million pounds of wheat to get just one pound of octacosanol.

What is Wheat Germ?

The "germ" is the embryo of the wheat kernel. It contains vitamins, minerals, sex hormones, vitamin E, various polyunsaturated fats and oils.

The oil contains the octacosanol, a light tan, waxy substance.

During early experiments it was found that animals deprived of the factors in wheat germ oil became infertile or lost their reproductive efficiency. The infertility was linked to vitamin E. Later experiments link the problem to octacosanol instead.

Octacosanol may act as an aphrodisiac. It steps up production of semen in men and provides the extra energy needed for renewed passion. It is possible that octacosanol stimulates the pituitary gland, which controls almost everything that happens in the body.

Agility, total reaction time, and mental acuity can be helped by this remarkable natural substance that can relax muscles at the same time that it steps up reflexes. It gives you energy without resorting to the use of artificial stimulants.

Availability: Octacosanol can be found at most health food stores and drugstores.

Dosage: You'll find soft–gel capsules with amounts from 375 mcg to 3000 mcg, or even higher. Depending on your own needs, take one capsule three times a day with meals.

Fructose

Fructose is a sugar in use since 1874 for its special metabolic properties. Many Europeans and Americans use it as an alternative to table sugar (sucrose).

Fructose is sweeter than ordinary sugar and sweeter than honey. Therefore, a smaller quantity can be consumed to get the same taste.

It appears that some fructose is utilized by the body for energy purposes *without the requirement of insulin*. The amount of fructose that can be utilized without insulin depends on a great many factors and varies with the individual, but, the fact that some fructose can be utilized for energy without insulin is a definite advantage to the body.

The fructose that does not enter the bloodstream for energy use is stored in the liver, partially as glycogen. This glycogen will, at a later time, be *slowly* converted to glucose and will enter the bloodstream in an orderly time–delayed sequence. This portion will require insulin but does not initiate the frantic release of insulin from the pancreas that sucrose does.

O.K.—So What Does This Have To Do with Me and My Diet?

Most people love sweets.

It's one of the factors that puts weight on in the first place. Sugar in your coffee, sugar in your tea, cakes, candies, ice cream, sugary cereals— does this hit home with you?

That you can use less fructose than sugar, that fructose is partially insulin–independent, and that fructose converted into glucose will be slowly released into the bloodstream *avoids* the massive "insulin dump" (that causes you to feel super–tired and emotionally "let down") that usually comes from the use of sugar as a sweetener. This enables those individuals with a sweet tooth and, those individuals with sugar–related diseases, to utilize fructose while minimizing fluctuations in both high and low sugar levels.

But Sugar, Table Sugar That Is, Gives Me Energy

You're fooling yourself to get a sugar–fix.

An orange is a better energizer than a candy bar.

You don't belive it?

Here's the way it works.

Chew on a candy bar and you get an almost instant glucose high. But, the pancreas opens the flood gates and insulin spills into the bloodstream in response to the sugar. The insulin drives the sugar into the cells, then hunts all over the bloodstream for any leftover sugar. This hunt drives glucose levels down below where they were before you ate the candy bar. Your muscles now get less food and you feel more tired than before.

Eating fructose saves muscle glycogen, but eating regular sugar depletes it.

Fructose takes longer to get into the body's bloodstream, but doesn't need insulin to be made available to the muscles.

As said before, many people use table sugar to satisfy their craving for sweets. But sugar programs the body to store fat. Also, sugar has been linked to a number of diseases.

Regular consumption of fructose does not raise serum cholesterol or triglyceride levels.

Fructose does not contribute to dental caries.

Our bodies recognize fructose because fructose is the name for fruit sugar, the same sweetener that is found in apples, pears, strawberries, melons, and so on.

Availability: Fructose is available in health food stores and in supermarkets.

Dosage: Replace table sugar with a bowl of fructose, but use less of the fructose to get the same sweetness.

Cook and bake with it, replacing the sugar in your favorite recipes.

There are even fructose tablets on the market when you feel you must have a sweet taste in your mouth.

Look for diet aids containing fructose, because the little bit that is present will give you an energy lift when your calorie–cutting diet tends to make you feel a little down in the mouth.

Get natural fructose the way nature intended. Eat more fruit instead of candy bars.

Have an apple or a pear during your mid–morning and mid–afternoon break.

Look for fructose–sweetened foods instead of sugary foods. You'll be amazed at the number of calories saved!

Alpha–Ketogluterate

This is a strange–sounding substance that you might have trouble finding. It will probably be in combination with vitamin B–6 (pyridoxine) or in some other vitamin and mineral formula.

It helps to keep your energy up and your exercise level higher than you're used to.

Availability: It's a plus in a diet formula but don't worry if you don't find it. It'll take a while for the diet world to catch on to its potential. Try health food stores.

Dosage: Follow directions on package.

Vitamin B–15 (?)

Why the question mark? Because it's not a vitamin!

It is a natural substance, but the definition of a vitamin includes the facts that it has to be essential to human nutrition and, if it is lacking, a deficiency disease can be attributed to it.

So, B–15 is not a vitamin. Let's call it an accessory nutrient.

What Does It Do?

Principally, it increases both the supply of oxygen in the blood and its uptake into the body's tissues.

The Russians have done the most research on B–15. They say it is involved in protein synthesis, energy transport, that it stimulates the immune response, regulates the blood level of steroids and speeds recovery from fatigue.

Dr. Robert Atkins recommends B–15 to the weary in *Dr. Atkins' Super Energy Diet*. He uses it when none of the other vitamins work. He says that B–15 can turn a person's energy picture around surprisingly.

Substances that prevent fatty infiltration and promote fat transport within the body are called liptropic agents. Among such agents are the vitamins folic acid and B–12, plus the amino acids choline, methionine, and the digester betaine. Add B–15 to that list.

When minks were fed a diet that normally produces a fatty liver, but were also protected with B–15 supplement, it was found that fat transport from the liver increased, fat metabolism was increased, and total metabolism was increased.

Availability: Natural sources include liver, seeds, rice, and whole grains. The nutrient is also available in health food stores and some drugstores.

Dosage: Dr. Lutz of the Institute of Preventive Medicine has recommended a dose of 50 mg to 150 mg a day.

According to the FDA, B–15 is a supplement when it is used by itself and not in combination with any other substance. It does not recognize its use for any other purpose.

Guarana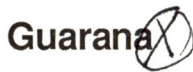

Commercially available weight–reduction products contain guarana as one of the ingredients.

It is found combined with glucomannan, and the advertisements indicate that the ingredients in guarana have the same chemical makeup as caffeine and cocaine, but can be used for weight reduction without any of the side effects of these drugs.

That may not be entirely true.

Guarana is the dried paste made from the crushed seeds of Paullinia cupana or Paullinia sorbilis. The plant is a shrub, native to Brazil. The seeds are collected and dry–roasted over a fire. Then the kernels are ground to a paste with cassava and molded into cylindrical sticks, which are then dried in the sun.

Although the stems, leaves, and roots are used as fish–killing potions in Central and South America, in Africa these are used to treat dysentery and as an aphrodisiac.

Guarana contains from 3 to 5 percent caffeine, but no cocaine. The appetite–suppressant effect is related to its caffeine content.

There are no published reports describing toxicity from guarana, but if you are sensitive to caffeine, use caution.

Many diet products found in drugstores combine caffeine with propanolamine.

Availability: Found in 15 mg tablets or capsules in health food stores and drugstores.

Dosage: Follow manufacturer's instructions.

Herbal Fat Fighters

Many companies offer herbal combinations that have been taken from folklore.

One such contains the following: glucomannan, chickweed, burdock root, chia seed, psyllium seed, and celery seed.

Because such formulas contain a large amount of fiber, they swell and expand in the stomach—providing they are taken with sufficient water.

It is said that in order to reduce the caloric density of the usual diet, you must provide extra volume to the stomach, promote the feeling of fullness, and slow the rate at which calories can be ingested.

These formulas also contribute to regularity by speeding the transit time of food throughout the body. By speeding up the transit time, mixtures such as the above help to decrease the absorption of dietary cholesterol.

Along with this concept must go diet!

Absolutely no junk food is to be eaten. Highly refined sugar foods throw the metabolism off and undermine all your good efforts.

Lecithin

Maybe after you've used it you'll call it "less–i–thin."

Lecithin is found in egg yolks and in some vegetable oils, but mostly it is found in soybean oil.

It's part of every single cell in your body, and its greatest concentration is in the brain. About 17 to 20 percent of the brain is made from lecithin.

But What Can It Do for Your Body, You Ask

I'll answer that question first so you'll want to keep reading about this marvelous natural substance; then I'll tell you more about all of the things it can do for you!

Lecithin is an emulsifier.

It's used in the manufacture of chocolate, for example.

It keeps the chocolate liquid, and thus keeps it moving.

Lecithin does the same thing for your fat—keeps it moving, moving right off you.

It's also a natural diuretic and an effective cholesterol–reducer.

In addition, it's the source of two of the hardest–to–find B–vitamins: choline and inositol. And it's loaded with sexy vitamin E.

Okay, I'll Listen to the Whole Lecithin Story

For thousands of years (even before 1,000 B. C.), the people of China have regarded the soybean as an extraordinary substance. One of the reasons for its reputation is that it includes all of the nutritional requirements for the human diet. No other food is as rich in the protein nutrients that are needed for energy, heat, and tissue repair.

The Chinese consider the soybean a perfect food. It is the only vegetable that is almost identical to the protein composition in animal food. It is called "the vegetable cow," and "the meat of the soil." It is high in protein (11 percent), low in fat (6 percent), with abundant amounts of vitamins A, B, C, and E, plus minerals and other trace elements.

Soybeans also contain twenty-two amino acids, which makes a meal of tofu (the way most Americans eat soybeans) very healthful and the easiest meal to digest.

Lecithin, a principal component of soybeans, is from the Greek (lekithos), literally meaning "egg yolk." But, lecithin is emerging not only as the great new hope in the treatment of many conditions, including obesity, but also for its ability to build up and release a neurotransmitter called acetylcholine.

Without acetylcholine, our ability to think, remember, and control our muscles goes haywire.

One major function of lecithin (also called phosphatidyl choline) is to supply choline in the diet. Choline is an important B-vitamin with the property of breaking down fat deposits in the body.

This property is used for the treatment of atherosclerosis (fat deposits in the walls of the arteries) and other problems caused by fat accumulation.

Choline is an essential ingredient of the nerve fluid acetylcholine, which is needed to connect nerve cells so that impulses can be transmitted from one nerve cell to another. Acetylcholine also bridges the gap (or synapse) between a nerve cell and a muscle cell. It is the fuel required for the nervous system to function properly and is essential for proper brain function.

Choline is distributed throughout our body in the blood and comes either from the food we eat, mostly as phosphatidyl choline, or from its manufacture in the liver. Our bodies do not manufacture enough choline, so we have to rely on getting it from our food or from supplements.

Availability: Usually at health food stores or drugstores.

Dosage: You can buy lecithin in granule or powder form to be mixed with food, or you can get capsules (1200 mg) or even chewable tablets with a nice vanilla taste (also 1200 mg).

Try taking two capsules, or chewing two tablets, after each meal.

A New Weigh

"Fat" is an ugly word in most vocabularies. However, fat serves an important purpose and the body needs an adequate amount.

So it's not fat but *excess fat* that is the problem.

Let's try to understand how fat, both necessary and excessive fat, is formed in the body. The food we eat supplies refined and complex carbohydrates. These are converted into glucose or other simple sugars in the small intestine, and then travel to the liver via the bloodstream. If blood–sugar levels are low, the liver releases all of the glucose to be circulated to all of the body tissues that require it for the production of body energy.

If blood–sugar levels are normal or above normal, the glucose may be converted in the liver into triglycerides, and eventually put into fat cells. Or, insulin may facilitate entry into the fat cell where the glucose will be converted into triglycerides and stored.

As discussed earlier, Brown Fat, also known as brown adipose tissue (BAT) is the desired kind of fat. White Fat, in excess, is undesirable. The difference between White Fat and Brown Fat is that White Fat acts primarily as insulation, fuel, and a protective layer for glands and organs.

On the other hand, Brown Fat actually produces heat, and, by doing so, burns calories. Brown Fat burns White Fat to produce heat.

Where Is Brown Fat Found in the Body?

It is found between the shoulder blades, behind the sternum, surrounding the kidneys and aorta, and around the muscles and blood vessels of the neck, where it gives direct warmth to the main flow of the circulation. When the skin temperature drops, Brown Fat burns triglycerides to restore the temperature to an even keel.

How Does BAT Affect Obesity?

It may be an answer to the question why, under similar circumstances, some people gain weight while others don't. As I have stated, *it is possible that people who gain weight rapidly have larger amounts of regular fat (White Fat), while those who don't gain weight easily have larger amounts of Brown Fat.*

Where Is White Fat Found in the Body?

Most White Fat is found beneath the skin. It is also stored in fat cells, between muscles, around the kidneys and other organs. It is also partially responsible for giving women their "figures."

Brown Fat usually makes up less than 1 percent of the total weight of the average human, although hibernating animals have considerably more.

White Fat is primarily a storage site for fatty acids that are released on demand, as when the stress response is triggered ("fight or flight").

Brown Fat reacts to activation of the sympathetic nervous system, and there are some foods that are able to increase that system's activity. When the sympathetic nervous system is activated, it releases the neurotransmitter norepinephrine. Foods that contain the amino acid tyramine facilitate its release, which then activates the Brown Fat.

Do Not Overdo These Foods

Eat them in moderation. If you suffer from migraine headaches, *avoid them*! If you take a prescription drug called MAO, *avoid them*!

Foods and Beverages That Contain Tyramine

Wine
Sherry
Champagne
Red wine
Chianti
Concord

Seafood
Salted herring
Pickled herring
Shell fish

Fruits and Vegetables
Banana
Plum
Avocado
Pineapple
Lemon
Tangerine
Tomato
Potato
Spinach
Eggplant

Fermented Products
Sauerkraut
Soy sauce
Vinegar

Cheeses
Brie
Herve
Roquefort
Edam
Gruyere
Limburger
Brick
Swiss
American
Camembert
Bruxellas
Blue
Maredsons
Cheddar
Gouda
Munster
Romano

Cool temperatures in the range of 65 or 66 degrees Fahrenheit are thought to activate Brown Fat. You need to be cold, but not cold enough to shiver. If you shiver, then the activity in the Brown Fat will decrease.

Exercises that do not increase body temperature will cause an increase in Brown Fat. Try swimming in luke–warm water.

We need some White Fat and as much Brown Fat as possible. See what you can do about it!

Crash Diets—If You Absolutely Must Lose a Few Pounds

These diets are not intended for long–term use, but just if you have to lose from six to ten pounds in a hurry.

If you have to get into that dress or that pair of pants, try these—but not if you want to lose a lot of weight and *keep it off*.

Take a good vitamin and mineral formula at least twice a day, and some fiber tablets with a full glass of water before meals.

Seven–Day Crash Plan

First Day

BREAKFAST:
Scrambled egg (use non–stick pan and Pam)
Whole wheat or bran muffin
Herbal tea (no sugar)

LUNCH:
Broiled hamburger on half a bun
Lettuce and tomato salad with lemon juice
Melon wedge
Herbal tea

SUPPER:
Broiled shrimp (4 ounces)
Small baked potato
Green salad with lemon juice
Small baked apple
Herbal tea

SNACK:
Apple
Club soda with lime juice

Second Day

BREAKFAST:
One medium orange
1/2 cup cooked oatmeal (sweetened with apple juice)
1/2 cup skim milk
Herbal tea

LUNCH:
1 cup clear broth
Green salad of cucumbers, beansprouts, watercress, lettuce
Cheddar cheese sandwich on whole wheat bread
Herbal tea

DINNER:
Low–salt tomato juice
Mixed salad with added green pepper
Roasted chicken without skin (3 ounces)
1 cup steamed broccoli
Herbal tea

SNACK:
1/2 cup unsweetened pineapple

Third Day

BREAKFAST:
Western omelet (use non–stick pan and Pam)
2 slices whole wheat bread (may be toasted)
Herbal tea

LUNCH:
Seafood salad of lettuce, tomatoes, and 4 broiled shrimp
Lemon–juice dressing
1 slice whole wheat bread
Herbal tea

DINNER:
Mixed green salad
Broiled sirloin steak (trimmed of fat) with sliced onions and mush-
    rooms (steak to be as close to 4 ounces as possible, after trimming)
1/2 cup steamed carrots and peas

Angel food cake (1–inch slice)
Herbal tea

SNACK:
1 cup fresh fruit salad

Fourth Day

BREAKFAST:
Medium orange
1 shredded wheat biscuit
1/2 cup skim milk
Herbal tea

LUNCH:

Salad of shredded apples, cabbage, carrots
Sliced turkey or chicken (without skin)
1 slice whole wheat bread (or toast)
Melon wedge
Herbal tea

DINNER:
Salad of lettuce, tomato, peppers, zucchini with dressing of lemon
    juice or apple cider vinegar
Broiled fillet of sole (4 ounces)
Steamed asparagus
Herbal tea

SNACK:
Fresh fruit, your choice

Fifth Day

BREAKFAST:
6 stewed prunes
Whole wheat muffin
1 pat butter
Herbal tea

LUNCH:
Lettuce and tomato salad
1 cup clear broth
Swiss cheese sandwich on whole wheat bread
Herbal tea

DINNER:
Green salad
2 small broiled lamb chops
1/2 cup steamed carrots or peas
Angel food cake (1–inch slice)
Herbal tea

SNACK:
1 cup fresh fruit salad

Sixth Day

BREAKFAST:
1/2 grapefruit
1 slice French toast
Herbal tea

LUNCH:
Mixed green salad
Tuna sandwich on whole wheat bread
Melon wedge
Herbal tea

DINNER:
Low–salt tomato juice
Mixed green salad
Broiled or roasted chicken without skin (3 ounces)
1/2 cup Brussels sprouts
Herbal tea

SNACK:
Medium apple

Seventh Day

BREAKFAST:
1/2 cup cooked oatmeal (sweetened with apple juice)
1/2 cup skim milk
1 slice whole wheat toast with a dab of butter
Herbal tea

LUNCH:
Chef's salad of 3 ounces cubed chicken, plus cucumbers, lettuce, to-
    matoes, and radishes, with dressing of lemon juice or apple cider
    vinegar
Small baked apple
Herbal tea

DINNER:
Mixed green salad
Choice of 4 ounces salmon or swordfish
1/2 cup steamed carrots
Small baked potato
Herbal tea

SNACK:
1 cup mixed fruit

Cutting Down on Calories
Is Easier Than You Think

You don't want to jump into a 1200–calorie routine all at once. You'll just activate Diet Panic and Diet Stress, and they'll work against you. What you really should do is ease into your food–reduction program slowly. Take your time and lower the calorie count week by week, losing 500 calories to 1,000 calories over a period of time. In that way you will keep Diet Panic and Diet Stress under control.

Remember to keep well–stocked with vitamins and minerals, and keep your belly happy with fiber.

You don't have to memorize all of the foods you eat with the number of calories they contain. The group listings that follow will give you a good approximation, and it covers most average American choices in the diet area. For example:

BREAKFAST:

Cooked whole grain cereal
1/2 cup whole milk
1 slice whole–grain bread
Herbal tea

LUNCH:

2 ounces white meat turkey
1 cup mixed carrots and green beans
1 baked potato
Herbal tea

SUPPER:

2 hard–boiled eggs
1 slice whole–grain bread
Lettuce and tomato salad
1 cup blueberries

This menu provides a total calorie count of only 830 calories, leaving room for reasonable snacks between meals and at bedtime.

Although this is a calorie–restricted program, it's not one that will give the average dieter too much trouble. By looking over the chart, and figuring what you like to eat and what you hate to eat, you'll find it easy to begin to judge other foods by comparing them to the chart.

It would be difficult to eat more than 2,000 calories if you selected only from the foods shown here.

Group One—Serving size 1 cup—average 35 calories

Asparagus	Cauliflower	Lettuce
Green beans	Celery	Mushrooms
Broccoli	Cucumber	Green peppers
Cabbage	Eggplant	Radishes

Group Two—Serving size 1 cup—average 45 calories

Artichokes	Lima beans	Peas
Bean sprouts	Rutabagas	Squash
Beets	Turnips	Baked potato
Carrots	Brussels sprouts	

Group Three—Serving size 1 cup—average 80 calories

Apple (fresh)	Cantaloupe	Plums (fresh)
Blackberries (unsweetened)	Cherries (fresh)	Strawberries (unsweetened)
Blueberries (unsweetened)	Honeydew melon	Watermelon
Boysenberries (unsweetened)	Orange Huckleberries (unsweetened)	

Group Four—Serving size as indicated—average 75 calories

Whole–grain bread (1 slice)	Granola or whole-grain dry cereal (1/2 cup)	Popcorn (1–1/2 cups)
Cooked whole–grain cereal (1/2 cup)		

Group Five—Serving size 2 ounces—average 150 calories

Beef	Eggs	Fish
Lamb	Turkey	Natural cheeses
Chicken	Liver	Cottage cheese

Group Six—Serving size as indicated—average 85 calories

Avocado (1/2)	Salad dressing (2 tbsp)	Skim milk (1 cup)
Butter (2 tsp)	Whole milk (1/2 cup)	Unflavored yogurt (1/2 cup)

The Basic Points of Some Recognized Diet Plans

If you go on any of these diets, make sure that you take a good vitamin/mineral supplement at least once a day.

Dr. Johnson's Pound–a–Week Diet

Dr. Harry Johnson, of the Life Extension Institute, tells his people not to change their diets or regular eating habits, but to cut 500 calories a day from their daily consumption.

Since 3500 calories add up to one pound of stored fat, you should lose one pound a week.

Cut on your intake of bread, sugar, sweets, and desserts rather than on fruits, vegetables, and meat.

The High–Protein, Low–Carbohydrate Diet

This is an eat–all–you–want diet, providing you eat certain foods. Eat all you want of eggs, cottage cheese, meat, poultry, and fish. Don't eat cold cuts, sausage, sugar, or starch. Do eat two small green salads daily. Do eat up to four ounces of cheese daily. Don't eat any carbohydrates at all for the first ten days. (This is not a diet you will stay on for an indefinite period of time. Just long enough to lose six to ten pounds.)

Feed Your Ideal Weight

This diet was designed by medical advisors to AT & T. First, find your ideal weight according to a good chart that takes into account height and frame.

Then, multiply your ideal weight by 12.

This will give you the number of calories you can consume daily.

If you want to be 120 pounds, your daily ration is 120 x 12, or 1440 calories.

Since you will then be feeding your ideal weight and not your over-weight self, you will eventually lose all of the excess pounds.

The Ultimate Diet—Fasting

For those who can tolerate total deprivation, Dr. Allan Cott and many other physicians recommend fasting as the most effective "diet" of all.

You can drink plenty of water, but no tea, coffee, or caffeine–containing drinks.

It will be difficult at first, but hunger pangs will subside after the second day or so. Weight loss will be rapid—perhaps three pounds the first day.

However, because prolonged fasting burns up muscle tissue as well as fat, never fast for more than four to seven days in a row without being under the care of a physician.

If total abstinence is too difficult, you can go on a juice and bouillon fast. Take up to eight glasses of natural or unsweetened fruit or vegetable juice, or low–calorie bouillon each day, but no solid food.

COMMENT:

People should never fast if any of these conditions is known or suspected:

- Tumor
- Bleeding ulcer
- Cancer
- Cerebral disease
- Kidney disease
- Gout
- Liver or blood disease
- Recent heart trouble
- Active lung disease
- Diabetes

Here is a Suggested One–Day Juice–Fast:

7:30 A.M.	Drink the juice of one lemon mixed with 8 oz. of water
8:30	Drink a glass of fresh orange juice
9:30	Drink a glass of unsalted tomato juice
10:30	Make a cup of alfalfa tea and sip it
11:30	Drink a glass of fresh apple juice
12:30 P.M.	Drink eight ounces of water
1:30	Drink a glass of grape juice
4:30	Drink a glass of pineapple juice
5:30	Drink a glass of prune juice
6:30	Make a cup of peppermint tea and sip it
7:30	Drink a glass of grapefruit juice
8:30	Make a cup of chamomile tea and sip it
9:30	Go to bed

Briefly here are a few of the nutritional values you've had during your juice–fast:

9 gm protein
195 mg calcium
2620 IU vitamin A
365 mg vitamin C
35 mg B–complex

Don't get on the scales until the next morning!

The 555 Diet

The menu cannot be changed and it is a tough one.

BREAKFAST:
4 ounces unsweetened fruit juice
Coffee or tea, must not use cream or sugar

MID–MORNING:
1 glass skim milk

LUNCH:
1 egg, cooked without butter
Large helping of lettuce with lemon juice dressing

MID–AFTERNOON:
1 medium apple or banana

DINNER:
1 cup clear consomme or bouillon
3 ounces lean meat, fish, or skinless chicken
1/2 slice toast
Large lettuce salad with lemon juice dressing

This is reasonably well–balanced nutritionally, but it offers only 555 calories and is a tough diet to follow. I wouldn't recommend it for more than ten days at a time.

Nibble Diet

Put together on the table:

1 hard boiled egg
1/2 pound of sliced tomatoes
1/2 cup cottage cheese
2 thin slices of ham
1/2 ounce of hard cheese
1/4 pound of grapes

Then divide all of the food into six portions.
This is all you will be allowed to eat.

Seven–Day Grapefruit Diet

Get your self–control ready. You can lose up to five pounds in five days. You must have grapefruit before every meal.

Don't weigh yourself every day. Step on the scales the day before your diet begins; then stay off for the next seven days. Weigh yourself on the eighth day.

Don't eat any fruit except grapefruit and lemon.

Don't eat any milk, cheese, or cream.

Don't have any sauces thickened with flour or eggs.

Don't use chili sauce, ketchup, or mayonnaise.

Don't eat corn or beets.

Don't eat pudding, rice, potatoes, bread, or pasta.

Don't use any sugar.

This is your menu for the next seven days:

BREAKFAST:

1/2 grapefruit

2 hard–boiled eggs

Herb tea with lemon, or black coffee

LUNCH:

1/2 grapefruit

Meat or fish prepared any way you like it, as long as it is not made with a sauce

Green or raw–vegetable salad with apple cider vinegar or lemon juice dressing

Herb tea with lemon, or black coffee

DINNER:

1/2 grapefruit

Meat or fish cooked the way you like best, but no sauce

Green or yellow vegetable

Tea or black coffee

BEDTIME:

4 ounces unsweetened grapefruit juice

Make sure that you are taking a strong vitamin and mineral tablet morning and night to provide any missing nutrients. You'll notice that there are no suggested portions of either fish or meat. That's because you can have a good portion of either just as long as it is baked or broiled, grilled or even sauteed, but without any sauce when served.

This is not a diet you should stay on for any length of time. Seven to ten days ought to get you into that dress.

Sea–Vegetable Diet

For those who would like the weight–loss benefits of sea vegetables, but who do not want to take kelp tablets, the following recipes should be interesting.

Try using one of these dishes once daily. The ingredients are available from your supermarket or from your local health food store.

Sea–Vegetable Rolls

3 avocados
1/2 cabbage, chopped finely
2 cups alfalfa sprouts
2 tbsp lemon juice
1 package nori sheets

Mash avocados and mix in cabbage, sprouts, and lemon juice.
Cut nori sheets in half.
Spread mixture on sheets, roll and serve.

Wakame and Cabbage Salad

2 cups cabbage sprouts
2 cups cabbage, finely chopped
1/2 cup wakame, soaked for 15 minutes and then drained

Mix well together and serve with sesame dressing.

Sesame Dressing

Soak 1 cup sesame seeds in a jar overnight.
Pour off the water and rinse well, then add a little water to make a
    paste.
Pour over the salad and add your favorite vegetables if desired.

Sea Guacamole

2 avocados
2 tbsp. lemon juice
1 stalk celery, chopped
1 scallion
1 cup radish sprouts
1/2 cup dry dulse in small pieces

Mash avocados and mix well with the lemon juice.
Add vegetables and dulse.
Mix well and serve.

Sea–Vegetable Salad

1 cup arame
1 cup dulse
3 scallions
2 red peppers
4 mushrooms
1 small clove garlic
1/2 cup lemon juice

Soak arame for about ten minutes and then drain.
Rinse dulse three times and mix with the arame.
Dice peppers, mushrooms, and scallions. Mix together.
Mix garlic and lemon juice in a blender and pour over the sea
    vegetables.
Mix well.

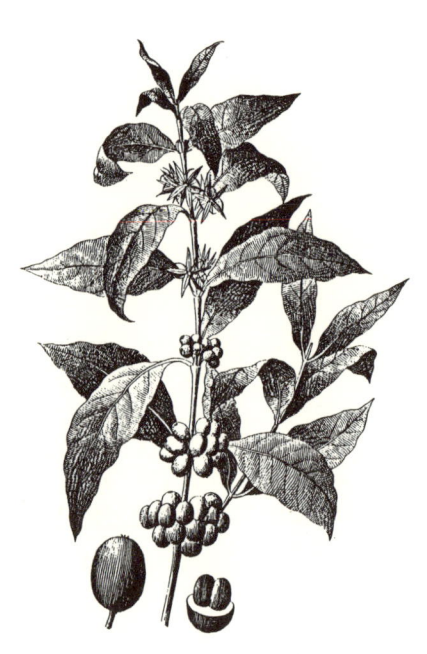

Contraindications

Before you go on any diet, make sure you can go on a diet without causing some problems. For most of us this means going to the doctor for a checkup.

Also, although the substances mentioned in this book are all natural and available without a prescription, there are some cautions to be observed.

Arginine and Ornithine

These are not to be used by people suffering from diabetes, ocular or brain herpes infection, pituitary dysfunction, or cancer.

GTF Chromium

Not to be used if you are allergic to yeast.

Fiber

Large amounts can interfere with absorption of nutrients from the food you eat. When using fiber, be sure you take supplemental vitamins and minerals.

L–carnitine

The use of D–carnitine or D–L carnitine has been associated with several severe side effects. Make sure that the substance you are using is pure L–carnitine.

L–phenylalanine

Do not use this supplement if you are taking a MAO inhibitor (some antidepressants). If you are not sure, ask your physician.

Do not use if you have cardiac arrhythmia, hypertension (high blood pressure), the genetic disease PKU, psychosis, or existing pigmented malignant melanoma type cancer, or if you have a violent temper.

Caution: if you are severely depressed, do not attempt to treat yourself, but do see a physician! There are many causes of depression, and your problem must be understood and dealt with accordingly.

L–tryptophan

Some individuals may be stimulated by the use of this amino acid instead of relaxed. Such individuals should not continue its use, since it is not readily apparent why this side effect occurs.

L–tyrosine

If you have a history of high blood pressure, you should monitor your pressure when using L–tyrosine. This is a matter of prudence.

Do not use L–tyrosine if you use MAO inhibitors, have cardiac arrhythmia, psychosis, preexisting malignant melanoma–type cancer, or if you have a violent temper.

Kelp

This should not be used to treat yourself for an underactive or overactive thyroid condition without the consent of your physician.

Drug Makers Hunt For Anti–Fat Pills

The huge profits that would result from an anti–fat pill sold by prescription have pharmaceutical companies working around the clock.

Researchers at such institutions as Massachusetts Institute of Technology (MIT) are looking at the link between brain chemistry and eating habits.

Dr. Jerrold G. Bernstein, director of MIT's clinical research center, and an expert on the effects of antidepressant drugs, has said that experiments have shown that you can alter the status of various important chemicals in the brain by what you eat or by taking a drug. He goes on to say that some drugs block the effects of chemicals in the brain that trigger appetite; others counteract depression that can lead to overeating.

Amphetamines (also known as "speed"), which have been used against obesity in the past did help to cut appetite, but they were also found to be highly addictive and caused personality changes. The prescriptions for amphetamine and its derivatives (benzedrine, dexadrine, and metamphetamine) were finally banned as a means of weight reduction.

MIT is working with an experimental drug called "dextrofenfluramine." It's supposed to help people who can't resist carbohydrate snacks.

Here's how MIT conducted the experiment: they put together a group of people with snacking problems and then set up vending machines. The vending machines were stocked with protein–rich foods such as delicious chicken, barbecued and designed to be as tasty as possible, lean corn beef (with and without a slice of sharp cheese), and other tempting protein dishes.

Next to the protein–vending machine was the carbohydrate–vending machine stocked with Snickers, pecan cookies, peanut cream patties, and other goodies (some even suggested by the test panel as being among their favorite snacks).

At first, almost 80 percent of the time, the test subjects snacked on the candies and cookies.

As they started taking the dextrofenfluramine, their tastes began to shift until they were eating the protein foods and cutting down on the carbohydrates.

As they did so, the pounds began to come off.

This research, and research being done at various clinics in the United States and abroad, is aimed at a new generation of anti–obesity drugs that will not be habit–forming and will not have serious side effects.

It's serious research with large rewards to the company that will come up with the right formula. The "fat" market is pegged at $200 million a year spent on various over–the–counter remedies, and that doesn't include all of the money paid out on exercise tapes, fat farms, and so on.

The MIT team holds the FDA investigational license to test dextrofenfluramine, but the drug is already being sold in France under the name "Isomeride."

It works by inducing the brain to produce a neurotransmitter called "serotonin," which, in turn, helps people reduce their craving for carbohydrates!

Doesn't that sound familiar? The first portion of this book dealt with nutritional manipulation of brain chemistry by using nutritional supplements!)

Another prescription drug that also works by stimulating the production of serotonin is called "fluoxetine." This drug was developed by the Eli Lilly Company. It was first put on the market as an antidepressant and, at that time, was named "Prozac."

Fluoxetine also prolongs the activity of serotonin, so that the effect is longer and people wanting to lose weight will not sink into a depressive state and go on an eating binge.

Since serotonin levels may exert their influence on cravings of all kinds (not limited to foods), it is possible that it could also be active against alcohol.

(I guess you've gotten the idea. Nutritional supplements can't be patented but drugs can!)

Conceptually, people may crave sweets and starches because of a low level of insulin (according to obesity specialists Richard and Judith Wurtman of MIT). This craving is in response to an effort to raise the insulin levels in the blood. Insulin helps an amino acid called "tryptophan" pass through the bloodstream into the brain area.

Tryptophan is an important building block in the manufacture of serotonin.

At the University of Washington, studies by Dr. Brad J. Wallum indicate that insulin may play a role in sending us the "stop eating" signal.

A shortage or absence of insulin, or a malfunction in how insulin is utilized in the body (see the discussion of GFT chromium in this book) may interfere with the signal, causing people to overeat. Animals reduced their food intake when insulin was administered directly into the brain area. This would be impossible for human subjects, but a synthetic hormone in pill form with the same action as insulin could be effective.

The Nova Pharmaceutical Company is researching a compound

called "NPC–168." It acts to block the effects of substances called "opiods" that attach to brain receptors to produce a morphine–like response.

These opiods, at least those that are found in the hypothalamus, appear to be stimulants to the appetite. If they are blocked, the desire to eat is also blocked. Animal tests have shown that NPC–168 caused reduction in food intake by 20 percent for almost twenty–four hours. The problem appears to be that it is only effective when given by injection.

Another group of drugs are being tested. They are called "thermogenics." These work by increasing the rate at which the body burns fat. While natural thermogenic compounds and methods do not appear to be harmful, synthetic compounds may increase the heart rate, leading to the risk of coronary problems.

St. Lukes–Roosevelt Hospital Center in New York City is investigating a compound called "chlorocitrate." It helps to produce weight loss by delaying the passage of food through the digestive system.

New York Hospital–Cornell Medical Center and St. Luke's Hospital Center are cooperating on a study of cholecystokinin (CCK), mentioned earlier in this book. It is called the "satiety hormone," and triggers the feeling of being satisfied no matter how little food is consumed.

Another substance called "bombesin," a peptide isolated from the skin of frogs, is being researched by Dr. Gregory Ervin at Duke University Medical Center. CCK and bombesin may join the ranks of prescription drugs being offered by physicians to help the obese.

Scientists consider obesity to be 20 percent or more over the ideal weight. Anything up to that obesity figure is considered "overweight." The table on the next page is based on the one used by Metropolitan Life for ages 25 to 59. The third figure in the column shows the approximate threshold of obesity.

Fat–fighting drugs are being prepared for promotion to the medical profession. In the meantime, it's up to you.

The perfect drug to control obesity would have to be able to curb appetite, be nonaddictive, have no potential for abuse, not be a stimulant, be reasonably long–acting, have no harmful effects on circulation, and have no other bad side effects.

According to Dr. Van Itallie, professor of medicine at Columbia University, the drug discussed in the first part of this section, dextrofenfluramine, meets this criteria.

This was quoted in an article appearing in the tabloid *National Enquirer*.

The drug appears to be superior to the amphetamines, but without the side effects that make amphetamines dangerous. The body can build up a tolerance to amphetamines, but dextrofenfluramine appears to maintain its effect for an indefinite period of time.

In a French study of 120 people, all of them more than 20 percent overweight, those given the new drug lost an average of fourteen pounds in three months, while a control group given a placebo tablet lost an average of only four pounds on the same diet.

All the people participating in the study lost weight according to Dr. Bernard Guy Grand, professor of internal medicine at Hotel Dieu Hospital in Paris, who conducted the study.

There were some side effects associated with its use, such as nausea and headaches, but not as many as when the progenitor, fenfluramine, was used. Dextrofenfluramine appeared to be twice as potent, with significantly fewer bad effects.

So, if you decline to use nutritional means, the pharmaceutical field will present its nominations shortly.

MEN

HEIGHT	SMALL		MEDIUM		LARGE	
5' 2"	125-131	157	128-138	166	135-148	178
5' 3"	127-133	160	130-140	168	137-151	181
5' 4"	129-135	162	132-143	172	139-155	186
5' 5"	131-137	164	134-146	175	141-159	191
5' 6"	133-140	168	137-149	179	144-163	196
5' 7"	135-143	172	140-152	182	147-167	200
5' 8"	137-146	175	143-155	186	150-171	205
5' 9"	139-149	179	146-158	190	153-175	210
5' 10"	141-152	182	149-161	193	156-179	215
5' 11"	144-155	186	152-165	198	159-183	220
6' 0"	147-159	191	155-169	203	163-187	224
6' 1"	150-163	196	159-173	208	167-192	230
6' 2"	153-167	200	162-177	212	171-197	236
6' 3"	157-171	205	166-182	218	176-202	242

WOMEN

HEIGHT	SMALL		MEDIUM		LARGE	
4' 9"	99-108	130	106-118	142	115-128	154
4' 10"	100-110	132	108-120	144	117-131	157
4' 11"	101-112	134	110-123	148	119-134	161
5' 0"	103-115	138	112-126	151	122-137	164
5' 1"	105-118	142	115-129	155	125-140	168
5' 2"	108-121	145	118-132	158	128-144	173
5' 3"	111-124	149	121-135	162	131-148	178
5' 4"	114-127	152	124-138	166	134-152	182
5' 5"	117-130	156	127-141	169	137-156	187
5' 6"	120-133	160	130-144	173	140-160	192
5' 7"	123-136	163	133-147	176	143-164	197
5' 8"	126-139	167	136-150	180	146-167	200
5' 9"	129-142	170	139-153	184	149-170	204
5' 10"	132-145	174	142-156	187	152-173	208

Source: Metropolitan Life Insurance Co. (1983)

Sampling of Scientific Investigations into Natural Substances

Chromium

Koslovsky, A.S., and others. "Effects of Diets High in Simple Sugars on Urinary Chromium Losses." *Metabolism* 35 (June 1986): 515–518.

High intakes of refined sugars may lead to marginal chromium deficiency. Strenuous exercise also increases urinary chromium excretion.

Octacosanol

Saint–John, M., and L. McNaughton. "Octacosanol Ingestion and Its Effects on Metabolic Responses to Submaximal Cycle Ergometry, Reaction Time." *International Clinical Nutrition Review* 6 (April/June 1986): 81–87.

Octacosanol supplementation in small doses can be effective as an ergogenic aid to improve certain aspects of physical performance.

Stomach Acid and Mental Stimulation

Feldman, M., and C. T. Richardson. "Role of Thought, Sight, Smell, and Taste of Food in the Cephalic Phase of Gastric Acid Secretion in Humans." *Gastroenterology* 90 (January 1986): 428–433.

Without tasting food, healthy volunteers were exposed to the smell and sight of food for thirty minutes. At other times they discussed appetizing food for thirty minutes without seeing or smelling any food. Measurements of gastric acid before, during, and after the stimulus period showed smell and sight of food increased acid production 23 to 33 percent. Food discussion produced a 66 percent increase.

L–carnitine

Keith, R.E. "Symptoms of Carnitine–like deficiency in a Trained Runner Taking Supplements." *Journal of the American Medical Association* 255 (7 March 1986): 1137.

L–carnitine, which is more expensive than the D–L form, could theoretically be of value for endurance. The author suggests that athletes avoid the use of D–L carnitine supplements.

Marconi, C., and others. "Effects of L–Carnitine Loading on the Aerobic and Anaerobic Performance of Endurance Athletes." *European Journal of Applied Physiology* 54 (1985): 131.

It is concluded that, in trained athletes, as a consequence of L–carnitine loading, V O 2 max is slightly but significantly raised, probably as a result of an activation of substrate flow through the TCA cycle, whereas the lipid contribution to metabolism in prolonged submaximal exercise remains unchanged.

(Comment: more energy from the same amount of fuel.)

L–carnitine acts as a carrier of fatty acid molecules into the mitochrondria of heart and skeletal muscle tissue, where fatty acid can be used by tissue cells as a source of energy.

L–carnitine is a natural substance, present in heart and skeletal muscle tissue. It is produced in the liver. A deficiency can occur if the liver fails to synthesize the substance, or if the carnitine is not transported from the liver to the heart or skeletal muscle.

A carnitine deficiency may be characterized by abnormal functioning of the muscle tissue. The body tends to accumulate fat that cannot be carried into muscle cells to be burned as an energy source. By supplying supplemental carnitine to correct a natural deficiency, the heart rate and force of contraction is increased. Carnitine has been used to relieve the symptoms of angina pectoris, the congenital disorder endocardial fibroelastosis and other heart disorders. It is also used for patients on renal dialysis. Studies are currently under way to evaluate its utility in other disease states.

Precautions—Large doses of carnitine have been associated with gastrointestinal symptoms, including diarrhea. L–carnitine is a natural substance. There are potentially dangerous impure forms of carnitine known as D–L carnitine.

(Comment: Look for the L–carnitine form of the supplement and never allow yourself to be talked into using the D–L form.)

Tryptophan, Obesity and Carbohydrates

Ashley, D.V.M., and others. "Evidence for Diminished Brain 5–Hydroxytryptamine Biosynthesis in Obese Diabetic and Non–Diabetic Humans." *American Journal of Clinical Nutrition* 42 (December 1985): 1240–1245.

Brain serotonin level may be impaired in obesity, suggesting a neurochemical basis for the association between appetite and mood in obese people. Abnormal carbohydrate craving may represent an attempt to normalize brain serotonin levels.

Herauef, E., and others. "Tryptophan Administration May Enhance Weight Loss by Some Moderately Obese Patients on a Protein–Sparing Modified Fast (PSMF) Diet."
Reprints of this study are available from Richard Wurtman, M. D., MIT, room E25–604, Cambridge, MA 02139.

Niacin (Vitamin B–3)

Knopp, R.H., M.D. and others. "Contrasting Effects of Unmodified and Time–Release Forms of Niacin on Lipoproteins in Hyperlipidemic Subjects: Clues to Mechanism of Action of Niacin." *Metabolism* 34 (July 1985): 642–650.
Niacin (vitamin B–3) has been used to help lower triglyceride levels and/or low density cholesterol levels in people with high levels of these lipoproteins. This article deals with a comparison of regular tablets of niacin and certain forms of niacin that have been treated to dissolve at different intervals throughout a time period. The latter is usually called time–release or time–disintegrating or other names that allude to a longer time span of release of the active ingredient.
According to the article, the regular tablets performed better than the time–release forms. They were much better when it came to decreasing the triglyceride and cholesterol amounts.
The dosage used during the experiments was very high (500 mg three times a day for one month, then 1,000 mg three times a day for five months) when compared to the RDA, so this regimen should not be attempted except with the help of your doctor. Flushing occurred with all patients taking the regular tablets and in 82 percent of the people taking the time–release form. Nausea, vomiting, diarrhea, fatigue, and decreased male sexual function were side effects found more frequently with the time–release form of the niacin.
Taking the niacin with meals can minimize the flushing reaction, or taking one aspirin tablet thirty minutes before taking niacin can help to cut down on side effects.

Dehydroepiandrosterone (DHEA)

Cleary, M.P., A. Shepherd, and B. Jenks. "Effect of Dehydroepiandrosterone on Growth in Lean and Obese Zucker Rats." *Journal of Nutrition* 114 (1984): 1242–1251.

Several studies were undertaken to determine the effects of DHEA on growth in Zucker rats. In experiment 1, three weeks of DHEA treatment in lean rats resulted in decreased body weight gain in comparison to control rats. In experiment 2, both lean and obese rats were treated with DHEA from six to twenty–one weeks of age. Significant decreases in body weight were found for both lean and obese DHEA–treated rats.

The food–efficiency ratio was significantly decreased in both DHEA–treated groups.

Significant decreases in parametrial and retroperitoneal fat pads were found in both lean and obese DHEA–treated rats. This was primarily attributed to a decrease in fat–cell numbers in lean rats and to decreases in both number and size of fat cells in obese rats.

In experiment 3, obese female rats were treated with DHEA from six to twenty–one weeks of age, followed by fifteen weeks with DHEA removed from the diet. Significantly more weight was gained by the rats previously treated than by the control group, but body weight remained far lower than in the control groups.

These data indicate that DHEA has an effect on altering body weight and body fat in lean and obese Zucker rats.

A considerable number of reports in the literature have suggested that supplementation with DHEA may be desirable for encouraging weight loss in the obese person.

The suggestions made are based on the work of A.G. Schwartz, who reported that the use of DHEA results in loss of adipose tissue in obese mice.

Current studies at the University of Minnesota have evaluated the effect of DHEA on growth and obesity in rats. The Minnesota research administered DHEA orally in food, whereas the research conducted by Schwartz used intravenous techniques.

The results indicate that DHEA has a positive effect on altering body weight and body fat and seems to encourage fat metabolism.

DHEA is a natural steroid metabolite found in the adrenal cortex. In supplemental use it can affect the manufacture of glucocorticoid hormones that help to regulate energy economy and fat metabolism.

Cleary, Shepherd, and Jenks postulate that the major action of DHEA is inhibition of the activity of glucose 6 phosphate dehydrogenase, resulting in decrease of lipid synthesis.

Although the amount of DHEA administered was high, no toxic effects were observed during or after the experiments.

Schwartz, A.G., G.C. Hard, L.L. Pashko, M. Abou–Gharbia, and D. Swern. "Dehydroepiandrosterone: An Anti–Obesity and Anti–Carcinogenic Agent." *Nutrition and Cancer* 3 (1981): 46–53.

Long–term treatment of female C3h–Avy/a(obese) and C3h–A/A(non–obese) mice with DHEA, an adrenal steroid found in subnormal levels in women predisposed to develop breast cancer, reduces weight gain without suppressing appetite, and significantly inhibits the development of spontaneous breast cancer.

This steroid also antagonizes the capacity of the tumor promoter, 12–tetradecanoylphorbol–13–acetate to stimulate 3–H–thymidine incorporation into mouse epidermis and in a cultured rat–kidney epithelial cell line.

Yen, A.T., Pearson, J.A., Donovan, V., June, M., Greenberg, M.M., "Prevention of Obesity in Avy/a mice by Dehydroepiandrosterone." *Lipids* 12 (1977): 409–413.

DHEA, a mammalian glucose–6–phosphate inhibitor, prevented Avy/a mice from becoming obese.

Decreased accumulation of triacetylglycerol accounted for a large portion of the weight difference between treated and control groups.

DHEA did not suppress appetite, had no apparent toxic effects at the doses used, and its weight–controlling effects were reversible upon withdrawal of treatment.

Schwartz, A.G., and R.H. Tannen. "Inhibition of 7,12–Dimethyl-benz[a]anthracene–and–Urethan–Induced Lung Tumor Formation in A/J Mice by Long–term Treatment with DHEA." *Carcinogenesis* 2 (1981): 1335–1337.

Migeon, C.J., A.R. Keller, B. Lawrence, and T.H. Shephard. "Dehydroepiandrosterone and Andristerosterone Levels in Human Plasma. Effect of Age and Sex: Day–to–Day Diurnal Variations." *Journal of Clinical Endocrinology* 17 (1957): 1051–1062.

Schwartz, A.G. "Inhibition of Spontaneous Breast Cancer Formation in Femal C3H (Avy/a) Mice by Long–Term Treatment with DHEA." *Cancer Research* 39 (March 1979): 1129–1132.

Oral DHEA was able to extend the life span of some laboratory animals by as much as 50 percent.

Oral DHEA prevented obesity in selected laboratory animals, and also prevented certain cancers induced into those animals.

The animals used were various strains of mice and rats. They received doses of DHEA in their regular food.

DHEA and its sulphurated derivatives are major adrenal secretory products in normal men and women. In humans, DHEA is the second most abundant steroid molecule. The only other steroid that is more abundant in the body is cholesterol. Although DHEA is classified as a hormone, there is some reservation as to whether this is a correct classification. Characteristically, hormones tend to be held in reserve in the gland that produces them, and they are then secreted into the blood stream when the body calls for them.

DHEA, which is manufactured in the adrenal glands, is not held there for the body's call. Instead, as soon as it is produced, it is released into the bloodstream to be used for cellular metabolism.

The levels of secreted DHEA decline greatly as the body ages. The body can lose 90 to 95 percent of the amount produced during the formative years by the time it reaches old age.

The decline of DHEA output corresponds with the increases in debilitating diseases (cancer, heart disease, obesity) that occur in later years. This has led to the possibility that DHEA supplementation might raise the amount in the body, thereby forestalling the appearance of aging and the appearance of these ailments.

Schwartz has noted that carcinogens require metabolic activation by NADPH–requiring oxidases (oxidative enzymes). NADPH is a coenzyme needed for the manufacture of these oxidative enzymes that change inert, but potentially carcinogenic, substances to true carcinogens. He postulates that DHEA inhibits carcinogen activation by lowering NADPH levels as a result of inhibition of another enzyme, glucose 6–phosphate dehydrogenase.

If DHEA can inhibit the enzyme activity, then it will inhibit the eventual production of carcinogens and will lower the risk of cancer.

In lower mammals, mice and rats to be precise, the anti carcinogenic effect of DHEA suggests that this steroid may have pharmacologic value in cancer prevention for humans.

It is unusual for young people to develop cancer. Perhaps one of the reasons is the abundance of DHEA circulating in their bodies.

Also, most teenagers and young adults up to the age of twenty–five have no difficulty maintaining a comfortable weight. DHEA is involved here, too, in the prevention of obesity.

DHEA and its metabolites are excreted through the urine.

Obese individuals excrete less DHEA and its metabolites than the non–obese. Urinary output of DHEA increases during weight loss.

Terence T. Yen, a researcher with Eli Lilly and Company in Indianapolis, Indiana, notes that these observations can lead to the hypothesis that DHEA may have a regulatory role in obesity.

The theory of how DHEA might prevent obesity is similar to the cancer–preventing theory.

The coenzyme NADPH is required for fatty–acid synthesis. The enzyme glucose–6–phosphate dehydrogenase is needed for the manufacture of NADPH. If DHEA inhibits this production, there will be less NADPH available to stimulate fatty acid production. Fewer dietary fats, carbohydrates, and proteins will be converted to storage fat. Instead, they will be converted to heat energy, or metabolized through other available non–fattening, biochemical pathways.

The theory has been tested on laboratory animals by Yen and others. The group receiving DHEA did not become obese, but the control group did. This happened even though both groups received the same amount of food.

As a weight–loss supplement, DHEA would prevent deposit of unnecessary storage fat. This would allow depletion of fatty–acid stores already held in the fat–storage cells of adipose tissues.

Theoretically, a person could lose existing weight by supplementing with a sufficient amount of DHEA.

Another noticed effect of supplementation was the unusual ability of animals to maintain youthful vitality and appearance. Not only did tested mice and rats remain slim and experience a much lower risk of cancer, but they also maintained good health and svelte bodies, with full vitality up to the moment of death.

The most striking feature of the DHEA research is that youth was maintained for quite a long time, with death coming at the end of a life span that was 50 percent beyond the normal life span for the test animals.

Testing on human beings is beginning now!

L–phenylalanine/Depression Treatment

Birkmayer, W., and others. "L–deprenyl plus L–phenylalanine in the Treatment of Depression." *Journal of Neurological Trans (cannot read manuscript)* 59 (January 1984) 81–87.

Unipolar depression was treated with the amino acid L–phenylalanine (250 mg per day) with the monoamine oxidase (MAO) inhibitor L–deprenyl (5–10 mg per day). Test was of 155 men and women. Improvement was noted in one to three weeks and culminated in full remission in 69 percent of the patients. Only 13 percent of the patients were not helped at all. The potent antidepressant action of this treatment is ascribed to accumulation of L–phenylalanine in the brain.

Sabelli, H.C., and others. "Clinical Studies on the Phenylalanine Hypothesis of Affective Disorder: Urine and Blood Phenylacetic Acid and Phenylalanine." *Journal of Clinical Psychiatry* 47 (February 1986): 66–70.

In forty patients with major depression, L–phenylalanine, the precursor of 2–phenylethylamine (PEA), given in gradually increasing doses up to 14 gr per day produced complete recovery in 27 percent and partial recovery in 50 percent with only minor side effects.

Stress–Induced Mineral Loss Might Be the Result of Strenuous Exercise

Anderson, R.A., M.M. Polansky, and N.A. Bryden. "Strenuous Running: Acute Effects of Chromium, Copper, Zinc, and Selected Clinical Variables in Urine and Serum of Male Runners." *Biological Trace Elements Research* 6 (1984): 327–336.

Strenuous aerobic exercise is associated with several therapeutic physiological and biochemical states. These include elevated HDL (the good blood fats), normalization of blood sugar, and reduced blood pressure. However, strenuous exercise also brings considerable stress to the body.

Stress can, however, produce changes that may not be what the individual wants.

Exercise can increase the demand for essential trace minerals such as chromium, copper, or zinc. It can also increase the excretion of those substances. If the dietary intake of them is borderline, the increased demand or increased excretion might necessitate an increase in the dietary amount needed.

Alterations in chromium and zinc are of particular interest, since these two minerals are involved in glucose metabolism. Factors that elevate glucose metabolism increase serum chromium. The mineral is not easily absorbed back into the system by the kidneys, so loss through the urine is increased.

In summary, exercise appears to significantly alter trace mineral concentrations and losses.

(Comment: this is of particular interest to dieters who have added strenuous exercise to their weight–loss program. The benefits of exercise are readily seen—loss of fat, normalization of blood sugar and blood pressure, and so on. However, it appears to be important to add a mineral supplement to your dietary regimen to insure a constant supply of those trace minerals necessary to prevent undesirable effects.)

Tyrosine and Stress

Reinstein, D., and others. "Dietary Tyrosine Suppresses the Rise in Plasma Corticosterone Following Acute Stress in Rats." *Life Sciences* 35 (1985): 2157.

Acute, uncontrollable stress increases norepinephrine (NE) turnover in a rat's brain and depletes it of NE. This diminishes the animal's subsequent tendency to explore a novel environment.

Pretreatment with tyrosine can reverse these adverse effects of stress, presumably by preventing the depletion of NE in the hypothalamus.

Various studies suggest that NE inhibits the release of adrenocorticotropic hormone (ACTH) by suppressing corticotropic releasing factor (CRF) secretion in the hypothalamus.

The conclusion is that tyrosine can protect against several adverse consequences of stress.

For three days, rats were fed a control diet containing tyrosine in food or by the use of supplements. They were then subjected to various stress–inducing mechanisms. Rats in the control group without tyrosine showed 50 percent more stress–reaction than the group getting the tyrosine.

Tyrosine prevented both biochemical and behavioral changes that occur from unavoidable stress. Depression in humans, which may be related to decreased brain norepinephrine and elevated plasma cortisol levels, might respond to supplemental tyrosine.

Pectin

Thomsen, L., A. Robertson, J. Wong, S. Lee, and C. Tasman–Jones. "Intra–caecal Short Chain Fatty Acids Are Altered by Dietary Pectin in the Rat." *Digestion* 29 (1984): 129–137.

In the bowel, the short chain fatty acid (SCFA) n–butyrate is produced by colon bacteria. This substance can alter cancer cells by accelerating their reproduction, altering their structure, and elevating some of their enzymes.

To determine the speed and effectiveness of dietary pectin in altering short chain fatty acids in the colon, researchers at the Department of Medicine, University of Aukland, New Zealand, did work on rats.

An experimental diet of 5 percent pectin and 17 percent fat was fed to the group, compared to the conventional diet of 3.3 percent crude fiber and 4 percent fat.

The experimental diet resulted in substantial reductions in caecal n–butyrate in pectin–fed rats when compared to rats fed the experimental diet without the pectin.

The results of the study show supplementation of dietary pectin to be an effective agent in modifying SCFA. Therefore, dietary fiber may play an important role in the health of the large bowel.

(Comment: pectin used to help transit time for weight loss has the added benefit of helping to protect the dieter against cancer of the bowel.)

Flourie, B., and others. "Effects of Increased Amounts of Pectin of Solid–Liquid Meal Digestion in a Healthy Man." *American Journal of Clinical Nutrition* 42 (1985): 495.

Pectin does not modify serum concentrations of secretin, cholecystokinin (CCK), vasoactive intestinal polypeptide, gastric inhibitory polypeptide, and somatostatin, but serum motilin and gastrin levels are below the control values after a high fiber meal.

(Comment: it may not make sense to you, but it's a plus for the use of pectin!)

Arginine Requirements

Visek, W.J. "Arginine Needs, Physiological State and Usual Diets: a Reevaluation." *Journal of Nutrition* 116 (January 1986) 36–46.

The usual American diet may provide barely sufficient quantities of arginine. Though often classed as a dispensable amino acid on the basis of growth and nitrogen balance data, enhancement of arginine intake may be beneficial in some circumstances.

Fructose

Levine, L., and others. "Fructose and Glucose Ingestion and Muscle Glycogen Use During Submaximal Exercise." *Journal of Applied Physiology* 55 (December 1983): 1767–1771.

When fructose is ingested before exercise, stable blood glucose and insulin levels are maintained and muscle glycogen is spared.

Dietary Fibers

Roos, J., and others. "Dietary Fiber Constituents of Selected Fruits and Vegetables. *Journal of the American Dietetic Association* (1985): 1111.

This study compared the dietary fiber, neutral detergent fiber, cellulose, hemicellulose, lignin, and pectin content of selected fruits and vegetables.

Apples were highest in cellulose, strawberries were highest in lignin, and oranges were highest in pectin.

With vegetables, green beans were highest in cellulose and hemicellulose, potatoes were highest in lignin, and carrots were highest in pectin.

Anderson, J. "Physiological and Metabolic Effects of Dietary Fiber." *Federal Procedures* 44 (1985): 2902.

William Beaumont noted the gastric effects of vegetable fiber and suggested that dietary fiber may provide health benefits. In the last decade, investigators documented the physiological effects on gastric emptying, intestinal nutrient absorption, and colon function. Increased fiber consumption and its effects, as pioneered by Beaumont's repetitive observations, should be undertaken to definitely establish guidelines.

Schneeman, B., and others. "Effects of Nutrients and Nonnutrients on Food Intake." *American Journal of Clinical Nutrition* 42 (1985): 966.

Protein, trypsin inhibitor, and fiber can alter food intake by several unique mechanisms, but there may also be some common mechanisms. For example, both poorly digested protein and fibers like guar gum and pectin lead to an accumulation of material in the small intestine. They appear to delay nutrient absorption, both in terms of the time–course of absorption and, within the intestine, the delayed rate of progress to more distal regions of the gut. These factors could contribute to reduction in food intake associated with ingestion of these substances.

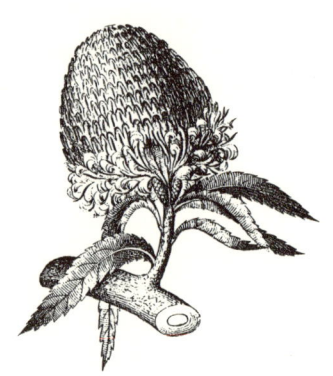

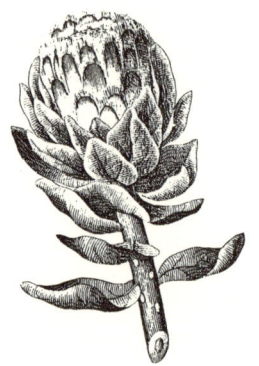

More Dietary News

Weight Lifting

The *Southern Medical Journal* tells us there's more to weight lifting than getting rid of flab. Weight lifting may increase the amount of *good* cholesterol (HDL) in the blood and thus help to prevent heart disease.

Researchers in West Virginia studied forty–five men with limited experience in lifting weights. After participating in a weight lifting program, the men experienced an increase in HDL. There also was a decrease in the *bad* cholesterol (LDL).

The study was done by the Department of Medicine and the Human Performance Laboratory, West Virginia University.

Crash Diets

In the *American Journal of Clinical Nutrition* we read that crash diets can hurt more than they can help.

A hospital–supervised crash diet of 400 calories a day, used by five obese women, although it contained all of the RDAs of all vitamins and minerals, resulted in muscle–cell deterioration after three weeks. Muscle cells couldn't contract and relax in a proper fashion because of an inability to utilize calcium. As a result, the women felt intense fatigue and a desire to do nothing more than rest.

Any crash diet of less than 800 to 1,000 calories a day can cause fatigue.

(Vitamins are not food. A person taking nothing but vitamins could starve to death. Vitamins help the body use food in a proper manner. They are not to be considered a substitute for food.)

Amino Acids for Depression

The mind affects the body; the body affects the mind. According to an article in *Neurotransmitter*, a large group of depressed patients who had not responded to conventional drug therapy were placed on a schedule of antidepressant drugs, plus the amino acid L–phenylalanine.

Some of the patients (102 of them) were given the combination of drug and amino acid by mouth, while another batch (53 patients) received their treatment intravenously.

In both groups 69 percent of the patients showed improvement in one to three weeks, resulting in full recovery from their depression.

Moderate improvement was noted in 21 percent of the patients who were treated orally, and in 11 percent of the patients given the medication by injection.

Only one in seven was not helped.

Because L–phenylalanine causes stimulating neurotransmitters to be released by the brain, some of the patients reported problems in getting to sleep at night. Others said they were a bit more tense and anxious. However, the combination of amino acid and drug worked where the drug alone had little use.

(It is possible that the side effects could have been avoided by substituting L–tyrosine for L–phenylalanine; however, the concept of combining drug and nutrient therapy is an exciting one.)

Amino acids help guard against depression say researchers from McGill University in Toronto, Canada, as reported in *Pharmacology, Biochemistry and Behavior*.

Tryptophan, as well as a combination of two other amino acids, L–phenylalanine and L–tyrosine, could help boost performance at work and guard against depression as measured on a multiple effect checklist.

A diet–induced depletion of tryptophan can lower mood as measured by self–report and task performance.

With the use of the amino acid there is a release of serotonin, a tryptophan–dependent neurochemical involved in depression. This chemical helps protect against the "blues."

The amino acids mentioned are usually available at health food or drugstores and are generally considered safe to use in the recommended doses. Asthmatics should consult with their doctors before using tryptophan because they may have a reduced ability to absorb it. This refers to asthmatics with endogenous (internally caused) asthma. Lower doses, such as 200 mg a day, have caused less reaction than higher doses (1200 mg a day). However, if you suffer from asthma, it would be wise to check first with your physician before you self–administer any dose.

Laxatives

If you take laxatives you are not alone. *Science Digest* reveals that one out of every ten Americans, twenty–two million or so, take them. But, what kind did you choose and what are you doing to your body by making it rely on them?

There's the overnight laxative. It needs stomach acid in order to work. This type may not, therefore, be the best choice for older people, who are often deficient in stomach acid.

Stimulant laxatives use the body's fluid to soften stools and make them easier to pass. Castor oil is one example. It may cause dehydration and loss of potassium and sodium.

Mineral oil, if used on a regular basis, can cause the loss of the oil-soluble vitamins A, E, D, and K.

So what's a person to do?

Eat fiber–rich foods, eat bran, all kinds of corn, oat, and wheat bran; eat carrots, mangoes, blueberries, and drink lots of water every day.

Regularity is a natural function of the body and the body will respond naturally to fiber and sufficient water. If necessary, fiber tablets or fiber cookies are available at health food stores. Fiber cookies contain 3 to 5 gm of fiber and don't taste bad. They can even be used as a snack or a sweet to end a meal. Look for a brand of fiber cookie that is made without sugar. There are even tablets made out of prunes if you don't like to have the real thing. When a natural solution is available, it doesn't pay to take a chemical.

Caffeine

In 1981, the *American Journal of Epidemiology* questioned some studies that linked caffeine with an increased risk of heart disease. What was true then is also true today. Caffeine does produce heart–rhythm abnormalities in some cardiac patients who are sensitive to caffeine. For this reason, heart patients or those at risk for heart disease should moderate their caffeine intake.

Caffeine is certainly not a modern phenomena. For well over one thousand years coffee beans, kola nuts, tea leaves, and cocoa beans have been used to provide an extra bit of energy. What is new is the awareness of the possible danger of too much caffeine. Everyone knows that coffee contains caffeine, but few know that a chocolate bar also contains the stimulant. For that matter, so do tea, cocoa, some carbonated beverages, and some drugs.

Caffeine directly stimulates the central nervous system. It helps to produce a wakeful state, and in large amounts can cause nervousness, hyperactivity, and a jittery sensation. It directly stimulates the heart, which causes the coronary arteries to dilate. Blood flow increases along with blood pressure and pulse rate.

In the brain, blood vessels constrict under the influence of caffeine, reducing the flow of cerebral blood. The muscle of the respiratory system and the gastrointestinal system relax, and output of urine increases.

However, caffeine also increases capacity for work, speed, and, in some cases, efficiency. Reaction time can be increased, as well as appreciation of sensory stimuli.

It's good to know all sides of a question. If you are not overly sensitive to it, a little caffeine may be helpful, while more than a little can be dangerous.

Barley and Oats

The Agricultural Research Service of the United States Department of Agriculture declares that barley and oats have cholesterol inhibitors, a triglyceride and a tocotrienol, which may decrease the risk of heart disease.

The inhibitors were identified by scientists of the Department of Agriculture and the University of Wisconsin. They say the substances affect the activity of enzymes that control the rate at which cholesterol is made and broken down into bile acids.

Additional research by James W. Anderson of the Veterans Administration Hospital at Lexington, Kentucky, showed that diabetic men who consumed about 100 gm of an oat bran fraction daily no longer needed shots of insulin to control their blood glucose.

At the present, although oats and barley are grown in the U. S., only about 7 percent of the oats grown and even less of the barley crop is consumed by humans!

Chromium

Adult Americans may not be achieving adequate chromium levels, says the USDA. A survey the department did of thirty–two persons showed that all of them consumed less than the minimum–suggested safe and adequate level of 50 mcg per day.

Also reported was a test of seventy–six adults, which showed that chromium may play a role in preventing hyperglycemia and hypoglycemia, and that physical stress causes rapid depletion of chromium levels.

L–phenylalanine

In the United States, obesity is a growing problem that cannot be defeated by any single method now known. In *Discover* magazine, February 1981, John Langone's article "Girth of a Nation" tells us that many studies are focusing on the role of the brain in obesity cases. For many years scientists have known that the hypothalamus plays an important role in weight gain. When the hypothalamus is destroyed in a rat, the rat becomes an obese overeater.

New evidence suggests that the hypothalamus is the control center for a chemical called cholecystokinin (CCK). It is produced in the brain and in the intestinal tract. It is believed to be the chemical that tells us when we have had enough to eat. Therefore, too much CCK may produce an undereater and too little CCK may produce an overeater.

In recent studies, the amino acid L–phenylalanine has been linked to the release of CCK. It is one of the essential amino acids found naturally in meats and milk.

In the brain, L–phenylalanine is turned into norepinephrine. Studies now under way seem to suggest that L–phenylalanine causes the release of CCK. For this reason, many researchers believe L–phenylalanine may be useful in the control of excessive weight gain.

(–)–Threo–chlorocitric Acid

A.C. Sullivan, R.W. Guthrie, and J. Triscari observe that pharmacological therapy for the obese patient currently focuses on reducing food intake, and anorectic agents continue to be useful as short–term adjuncts to weight–control programs.

Anorectic drugs that are utilized in the treatment of obesity produce their effects by interacting with central nervous systems involved in appetite control. However, current views on appetite regulation support the involvement of both central and peripheral components, which are integrated by metabolic processes. To date, relatively little attention has been directed to peripherally acting anorectic agents.

The report by Sullivan and his colleagues describes the anorectic activity of one such compound, (–)–threo–chlorocitric acid. This agent is an effective anorectic, which decreases appetite, leading to significant reductions in body fat in experimental animals. It is also devoid of central nervous system stimulatory activity and does not produce conditioned aversion behavior in rats. Furthermore, there is no evidence of the development of tolerance or rebound eating either during or after discontinuation of drug treatment as is seen with most centrally acting anorectic agents. The proposed site of action is the upper gastrointestinal tract.

Hydroxycitric Acid (Brindall Berry)

A.C. Sullivan and J. Triscari, in a paper entitled "Novel Pharmacological Approaches to the Treatment of Obesity," published by the Department of Biochemical Nutrition, Roche Research Center, state that obesity results when an imbalance occurs between intake and expenditure.

Hydroxycitric acid significantly reduced food consumption and additionally altered the metabolic flux of dietary nutrients by diverting carbohydrate and its metabolites from lipid biosynthesis in the liver even under pairfeeding conditions.

Oil of Evening Primrose and Gamma–Linolenic Acid (GLA)

At St. Thomas Hospital, London, England, in 1981, evening primrose oil was used to treat sixty–five women with severe cases of premenstrual syndrome.

The study reported that 61 percent of the women had complete relief from their symptoms, 23 percent reported partial relief and 15 percent reported no change.

One symptom, breast discomfort, was alleviated in more than 70 percent of the cases. Other common symptoms that improved were mood changes, anxiety and irritability, headaches, and fluid retention.

In 1982, research on benign breast disease (where the breast feels tender and lumps are present) was undertaken with seventy–two women at Ninewells Hospital, Dundee, Scotland. After three months of supplementation with evening primrose oil, both the tenderness and the lumpiness were relieved in a majority of the cases.

The Lancet, a British medical journal, has stated that in relation to obesity, EPO is thought to stimulate the activity of Brown Fat, a special tissue that burns calories to produce body heat. It also encourages an enzyme called sodium–potassium–ATPase, which is essential in the use of energy in the body.

Sodium–potassium–ATPase is said to use as much as 20 percent of the total energy (calories) available to the body.

In faulty immune system reactions, such as eczema and allergies, research conducted in England and reported in *The Lancet* in 1982 showed that sufferers of such diseases had normal amounts of linoleic acid in their blood, but were deficient in gamma–linolenic acid. EPO, which has naturally occurring GLA, bypasses the need for the Delta–6–desaturase enzyme in the first steps of the conversion of linoleic acid to gamma–linolenic acid.

Arthritis and Rheumatism in 1973 and *Clinical Immunology* in 1978 each reported that in relation to arthritis, animal studies have shown that PGE–1 can ease experimental arthritis in rats.

It can also activate T–lymphocytes, and control lysosomal enzyme release in humans—actions related to aiding symptoms of inflammation and faulty immune system reaction.

(Comment: there is much to be said for the use of GLA as a supplement, not only for its use to help control weight, but in a number of other situations.)

Fiber

Several articles have appeared recently on the subject of fiber in diet. In "Fiber and the Gut," published in the August, 1987, issue of *The American Journal of Medicine,* the author declares that fiber is truly one of the marvels of nature. A major contribution that has been made by the health food industry is the "rediscovery" of fiber. In the past five hundred years, civilization has been processing more and more of its food. One of the casualties has been dietary fiber. At the same time, incidences of colonic cancer, diverticulitis, gallstones, diabetes, atherosclerosis, and obesity have risen dramatically. There is widespread belief that the loss of fiber in the diet has had a definite effect on human health.

There are many examples in the scientific literature of the ability of fiber in the diet to regulate insulin release and hunger response. "How Fiber May Prevent Obesity; Promotion of Satiety and Prevention of Rebound Hypoglycemia," in *American Journal of Clinical Nutrition,* October, 1978, discusses this. In studies where people are given apple juice or whole apples, those who have the processed and fiberless apple juice experience a rise in insulin, resulting in a hypoglycemic rebound. Not only that, but the people who drink their apples are not as satisfied as those who eat their apples. Hunger satisfaction must have something to do with the amount of fiber eaten.

In an article entitled "Food Fiber as an Obstacle to Energy Intake," found in *The Lancet* (22 December 1973), one doctor suggests that fiber helps us cut down on the amount we eat in three ways. First, it displaces available nutrients from the diet. Second, it requires chewing, which cuts down on how fast we can eat. Chewing also promotes secretion of digestive juices that help fill the stomach and make us feel full. Third, fiber makes the small intestine less able to absorb. He concludes by saying, "The extreme commonness of obesity in Western countries may be related to the fact that most dietary carbohydrate is refined and fiber–depleted.

Thus, one successful method of weight control might include extra fiber to help fill the stomach with non–nutritive substance to keep us feeling full.

One other thing that fiber is general, and glucomannan in particular, are helpful for is control of diabetes. Two articles address this subject: "Treatment of Diabetes with Glucomannan," from *The Lancet* (May 5, 1979); and "'Devil's Tongue' Rx Cuts Sugar in Diabetics' Blood," published in *Medical Tribune* (April 25, 1979).

Dietary fiber has been used to successfully treat diabetes, often with a reduction in the dose of insulin. Glucomannan is a normal Japanese foodstuff taken in gelled form. It is an unabsorbable polysaccharide from the tubers of the amorphophallus plant, also called "Devil's Tongue." Dr. Matsuura, from the Department of Internal Medicine, Kobe University, has done a study on twenty adult–onset diabetics who took between 3.9 gm and 7.8 gm of glucomannan each day for four months. Patients who were using insulin were so well–maintained on the glucomannan that they were able to either reduce their insulin or switch to oral medication. Other researchers have also found that serum cholesterol decreased.

All in all, it looks good for fiber in the diet as a method of weight control. And glucomannan looks especially interesting.

Questions and Answers

I have kept a collection of questions I've been asked since people found that I was writing a book about diets. You may be interested in the questions and how I answered them.

Q. When should I eat?

A. Eat only when you are hungry. It sounds obvious, but many of us eat because the clock tells us to. Stop eating at a point when you feel you could eat a bit more. If you want to linger at the table for a little conversation, have a glass of herbal tea.

   Don't eat standing up. Eat slowly. Your brain needs time to get the message. Don't read or watch TV when you eat. You'll eat more than you want to. Buy small plates so the amount of food looks larger.

Q. Do I have to count calories if I want to lose weight?

A. Weight is a reflection of the energy balance in your body. If you take in more energy than you put out, the body will store it as fat. That doesn't mean you have to memorize the calorie content of all of the foods you eat. You know which foods are fattening and how much you should eat.

   Rather than count calories and alarm the body into storing anything you eat as fat, change the food you eat for foods that are high in nutrition and low in calories. Foods that contain a lot of fat are fattening!

   Proteins and carbohydrates have less fat and are less fattening. Sometimes you can substitute one food for another and cut calories almost automatically. Take a look at this list:

Instead of	Try
French fries	Baked potato
Mashed potatoes	Boiled potatoes
Candied yams	Baked yams
Creamed corn	Steamed corn
Creamed spinach	Spinach salad
Green beans almondine	Steamed green beans
Tomato juice	Whole tomato
Apple pie	Baked apple
Danish pastry	Raisin bread
French toast	Cinnamon toast

Instead of	Try
Chocolate cake	Pound cake
Fried chicken	Broiled chicken
Salisbury steak	Broiled hamburger
Scrambled egg	Poached egg
Whole milk	Skim milk
Cream cheese	Low–fat cottage cheese
Ice cream	Frozen yogurt

You can exercise your freedom of choice and choose the lower–calorie dish and still enjoy your meals.

Q. Is there a set amount of calories I should have daily when I am trying to lose weight?

A. That depends on your weight at the start. Your body will draw on its fat reserves when you take in fewer calories. Up to a point, it will burn off excess fat. If you gradually cut your caloric intake, your body will respond.

Don't crash diet unless you must lose a few pounds in a hurry!

One pound of fat equals about 3,500 calories. When you reduce your caloric intake by 3,500 calories and use up the same energy, you will lose one pound. If you reduce your caloric intake by 3,500 calories and increase your energy expenditure by exercising you will lose a little more than one pound

Although this doesn't sound like a lot of weight loss, consider that one pound a week adds up to a 52–pound weight loss by the end of a year.

Q. Some of my friends went on a 600 calorie diet. Should I try it?

A. What do those friends look like now? Have they really lost weight or are they fatter than ever? Remember what the body does if it thinks there is a famine!

Q. Are all fish low in calories?

A. We used to think so, but if you look at the following table you'll see that all fish are not fat–equal.

Fish Calories in 3–1/2 ounces—cooked

Bass	228
Bluefish	160
Cod, broiled	162
Croaker, baked	133
Eel	233
Fishsticks, frozen	176
Flounder, baked	202
Haddock, broiled	141

Herring, kippered	211
Mackerel, broiled	300
Pompano, broiled	284
Salmon, canned	203
Sardines, canned in oil	311
Trout	196
Tuna, canned in oil	288
Tuna, canned in water	127
Clams, raw	82
Crab, steamed	93
Lobster, canned	88
Oysters, raw	66
Scallops, steamed	112
Shrimp	80

This is a hard question to answer correctly because there's another issue involved. Healthful oils are found in fatty fish such as mackerel, salmon, sardines, and tuna. They are very good as potential building blocks for hormone–like substances called prostaglandins. I think I would rather have the fattier fish and exercise more.

Q. Am I fat because my parents were fat?

A. Obesity is both environmental and due to heredity. Studies show that children with normal–weight parents have a 15 percent chance of being fat, while if one parent is overweight the figure jumps to as high as 40 percent. If both parents are overweight, the percentage goes even higher.
While it is true that you may inherit a tendency to be fat, don't use it as an excuse to explain your increasing girth.

Q. My husband and I eat the same amount, but he doesn't seem to gain as much weight as I do.

A. Women seem to gain weight rapidly and keep on gaining weight, while most men, while they also gain weight, seem to level off after the age of 55.
It may be due to menopause, or it may be due to the fact that women are usually less active than men once the children have left the house. Women have more fat on their bodies than men do and need fewer calories to begin with. Nobody really has the answer to this one, so just cut down on your portion of food.

Q. How much food is a "portion"?

A. A half–cup of vegetables
Three–to–four ounces of fish, meat, or poultry
A glass of milk

One slice of bread

One apple or one orange

A half–cup of rice, noodles, or spaghetti

Or 1/2 the amount you ate when you were getting fat.

Q. Will a diuretic help me to lose weight?

A. It only appears to help. While it is true you will weigh less after taking a diuretic, it is only a loss of water, and along with it, a loss of minerals. As soon as you drink a few glasses of water, the weight loss will disappear.

Q. What are some good snacks to eat?

A. Fresh fruits and vegetables, fruits in their own juice, small amounts of dried fruits, popcorn without butter, rice cakes, whole wheat raisin bread.

Q. When I eat out and limit my meal to a salad bar, can I stay on a low–fat diet?

A. It is possible if you're careful to stay away from bacon bits, croutons, prepared salad dressings, and the like. Choose salad greens, chopped vegetables such as carrots and green peppers, chick peas, mushrooms, and bean sprouts. Use vinegar or a squeeze of lemon for dressing.

Q. Will exercise help me to lose weight?

A. It will help you to lose weight, and it will also help maintain muscle tone and skin tone as the weight comes off.

Q. I eat more than I should due to nervousness and anxiety. Is there anything I can take to help me?

A. As long as your problems are not due to a physical condition, you can try to take some L–tryptophan (one tablet during the day). Or, see if you can find some capsules of inositol, one of the B–complex vitamins. They have a calming action.

Q. I've heard that caffeine can interfere with weight loss. I can't think straight unless I've had my morning coffee. What do you think?

A. Moderate amounts of coffee will have little to do with whether or not you lose weight. Some people find a cup of coffee in the morning gives them the pep to go out and exercise.

Q. What about artificial sweeteners?

A. One thing you have to agree with—they're not food and they can't benefit the body in any way. So why take them!

Q. How about diet pills?

A. The best medicine is the least medicine, particularly when the side effects can be dangerous. Many over–the–counter diet pills contain phenylpropanolamine (it looks like phenylalanine, an amino acid, but it is not the same). It causes the brain to produce appetite–sup-

pressing chemicals, but loses its effect after a short time. L–phenylalanine will do the same thing without losing its strength.

Q.   What about alcohol, some diets permit white wine?

A.   Alcohol has no place on any weight loss program. It adds calories,
and makes you hungrier and less careful about what you eat.

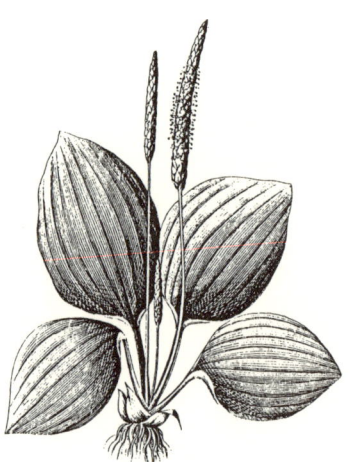

Epilogue

Just when I thought I had ended this book, a batch of new thoughts were dumped on my desk. It happens at the end of each book, and I should have expected it! Instead of putting them aside, however, and waiting for the "next" book, I'd rather share them with you at this time.

First, About a Possible Thyroid Condition

While it's true that almost all of the people who blame their obesity on the thyroid gland should blame their mouths instead, there are some people who do have thyroid problems. But, obesity is only one symptom of a malfunctioning thyroid.

And, it's not always able to be diagnosed through the regular blood tests administered by most doctors. A thyroid deficiency can lead to an astonishing and confusing set of symptoms. People suffering from a thyroid deficiency can experience coarsening hair, difficulty with breathing, skin problems, swollen feet, eczema, adult–onset acne, hoarseness, excessive or painful menstruation, poor memory, nervousness, brittle nails, depression, and headaches. The body is also subject to infection. But that's not all! According to Dr. Stephen Langer, M.D., in his book *Solved: The Riddle of Illness*, a thyroid deficiency has been linked to over one hundred known symptoms, including premenstrual syndrome (PMS).

Blood Tests Don't Tell the Whole Story?

Blood tests only measure thyroid hormone production. This means that the thyroid gland is either producing enough or not enough hormone. If it is not producing enough, the obvious solution is to supplement the hormone.

In many cases, however, there is enough thyroid hormone circulating in the blood. The problem is that the body is not using it efficiently. This condition is called subclinical hypothyroidism.

Is It a Common Disease?

It's not as common as a cold, but more common in these times than in the past. Thyroid hormones regulate oxygen consumption and energy flow, and the gland is uniquely susceptible to stress. In our modern world there is an overabundance of stress. There is also pollution–stress due to the assault of toxic chemicals in our food, air, and water.

How Can I Find Out Whether I Suffer from Subclinical Hypothyroidism?

You must see an M.D.

There is also a simple test to do before you see the doctor.

It is a simple and effective way to uncover hidden thyroid deficiency. It was discovered over thirty years ago by Dr. Broda D. Barnes. He found that a subnormal basal temperature (97.8 degrees or lower) is often correlated with hypothyroidism. The test is done as soon as you wake up in the morning.

Leave a regular thermometer near the bedside.

As soon as you wake, place the thermometer underneath your arm, in the armpit. Lie there for ten minutes.

Read the thermometer, and, if it is 97.8 degrees or lower, be sure to tell your doctor.

Can I Take Vitamins to Solve the Problem?

While iodine and tyrosine are helpful, as well as all of the other nutrients, it is likely that some form of thyroid medication will be needed.

But, don't blame your fat on your thyroid—chances are that your problem has nothing to do with your glands!

B1 and Meals Ruin Diets

Throw away your salt shaker.

Many health problems, including obesity, are related to excessive use of salt. Salt can interfere with the body's sodium–potassium balance, and the body will not be able to function correctly. Many people consume ten times or more salt than the body needs.

Most processed foods are highly salted.

If you have a water softener, the water you drink has a high sodium content.

Japanese foods are very high in salt (tamari, miso, shoyu).

Don't Go On, I Know Salt Is Bad for Me, but Food Is Tasteless Otherwise

I wouldn't talk about the problem if I didn't have a solution. Diet foods are usually bland and difficult to stick to, but there are ways to spice up any meal without resorting to salt.

For example:

Black Pepper—Add a generous grinding, a teaspoonful to main dishes before cooking. After roasting or broiling, the peppery strength is cut to a nice pungency.

Curry Powder—This makes rice delicious. It's very good when mixed with a little water and some dry mustard. Experiment a bit.

Crushed Red Chili Peppers—Use them in tomato or corn bread dishes.

Ginger—Buy it fresh, peel, and grate. Add it to chicken dishes. If you want to use the juice, cut off a piece of the root and extract the juice with a garlic press.

Flaked bell peppers, garlic, horseradish, and onion—They go with *any* meal. They'll even make the blandest cottage cheese come alive.

Lemon Peel—Grate a fresh lemon, and use on fish or with a salad.

Mushrooms—Dried or in flakes, these add a meaty taste to meatless dishes.

Mustard Powder—Mix with a little water and spread on grilled or broiled foods. Eliminates the need for any salt.

Paprika—This is a good source of vitamin C, and a light flavoring agent.

Seeds—Select a variety, such as poppy, caraway, celery, pumpkin, and sunflower. Use them whole or grind them up and add to meat loaf. Sprinkle them on a salad. The unique taste on salads will keep you from using salad dressing with its extra calories.

Make your own salt substitute. Grind up the following and store in a tightly closed jar:

1 tbsp dried, grated lemon or lime peel
2 tbsp black pepper
1 tsp finely grated, dried ginger
1 tsp powdered kelp
1 tsp grated fennel seed

Or, as a variation try this:

3 tbsp minced, dried onion
2 tbsp powdered mustard

2 tbsp powdered turmeric
1 pinch ground ginger
1/4 tsp cayenne pepper
2 tbsp dried, powdered lemon peel

Store in a tightly closed jar.

Consider the salt content of the food you eat. A large dill pickle contains about 1,900 mg of sodium, while a cucumber of the same size contains only 10 mg.

Laxatives and Cholesterol

Metamucil, a popular over–the–counter laxative has also proved to be effective in reducing moderately high levels of blood cholesterol, reports Dr. James Anderson, professor of medicine at the University of Kentucky.

Metamucil contains psyllium seed and the water–soluble fiber obtained from the hulls of the seed. "Metamucil" is the trade name of one product, but there are also other products which contain the same blond psyllium seed found in Metamucil.

In a recent study, test subjects who took Metamucil three times a day showed reduced blood cholesterol levels within two weeks, and their levels continued to drop for eight weeks. The average reduction was 15 percent.

Metamucil also selectively reduced low density lipoproteins (the dangerous ones) by 20 percent and decreased the ratio between high density lipoprotein and low density lipoprotein from 3.2 to 2.6

Dr. Anderson notes that if the results are sustained, the risk of coronary heart disease would be reduced about 30 percent.

Of course, the men being tested lost weight as well. If you took a laxative three times a day you'd lose weight too!

There is a danger to this concept. The passage of food through the stomach and the intestines can interfere with the absorption of nutrients. Metamucil is a fine product for people who have difficulty in staying regular. The usual dose of this product taken once a day will have little effect on the absorption of nutrients. Using it more than once a day without medical supervision may be dangerous to some people.

Chlorella—The Latest Fiber from Mother Nature's Watery Cabinet

I've written about spirulina, glucomannan, and other fiber substances and the way they can help you to lose weight. I have also introduced you to another one–celled algae with even more impressive qualities. Now I can tell you more about it!

The name of this micro–algae is chlorella. It measures perhaps 5 microns in diameter and has been on this planet about two–and–a–half billion years. That is since the Precambrian period.

This fresh–water plant is a bundle of nutritional assets. It gets its name from its high content of chlorophyll (the highest of any known plant).

In addition to chlorophyll, it also contains vitamins, minerals, nucleic acids, amino acids, enzymes, anti–infective agents, dietary fiber, and something "new" called chlorella growth factor (CGF).

If It's So Good, Why Haven't We Heard about It Before?

First, because it's so small that it had to wait for the microscope to be perfected. It was not until 1890 that a Dutch researcher, trying to discover why a certain pond had green water, located the tiny plant.

One of the differences between chlorella and other plants such as spirulina, is that chlorella has strong cell walls. The cell walls are one of the reasons chlorella is valuable.

About 60 percent of chlorella is protein and about 20 percent carbohydrates and lipids. The proteins contain all of the amino acids known to be essential for the nutrition of animals and humans. The only drawback is a low content of methionine.

The vitamins found in chlorella cells include: vitamin C, provitamin A, thiamin, riboflavin, pyridoxine, niacin, pantothenic acid, folic acid, vitamin B–12, biotin, choline, vitamin K, lipoic acid, inositol, and paraaminobenzoic acid. The minerals in chlorella include: phosphorus, potassium, magnesium, sulphur, iron, calcium, manganese, copper, zinc, and cobalt.

Such high nutrient content enables chlorella to be of potential benefit to Third World nations as a food source. It is also a promising supplement for weight control.

Imagine Being Able to Lose Weight and Protect Your Body at the Same Time!

One of the most exciting and rewarding areas in modern medicine is that of immunology. This is the study of the immune system and the mechanisms the body has evolved to fight off any invading organisms, such as bacteria, viruses, chemicals, or foreign proteins. B–cells fight against bacteria; T–cells are active against viruses and cancer; macrophages act against cancer, foreign proteins, and chemicals. Macrophages are large cells that are located in the liver, spleen, lymph nodes, thymus, lungs, abdominal cavity, blood, and joints. One of the ways used to fight disease is to use substances that stimulate the body's production of these macrophages. Interferon is a natural secretion of the body thought to be a macrophage stimulant.

In 1973, Kojima and Associates, a research group in Japan, demonstrated the immune–stimulating and detoxification power of chlorella. It appears that chlorella increases natural interferon production in the body.

Other experiments have also shown that the water–soluble injected extracts of chlorella called chlorellan is able to increase the activity of the body's macrophages. Another white blood cell (polymorphonuclear leukocyte) is also activated in a nonspecific way to act against other invading substances.

While the use of chlorella against disease is still in the experimental stage, and should not be used as a possible "cure," it's nice to know that an obesity fighter may also stimulate the immune system to keep you healthier!

What Else Can We Expect from This Algae?

For one thing, sustained energy, even on a low–calorie diet.

According to researchers H.V. Kolman and R. Schmidt, "The real benefits which fresh water microalgae can provide to modern man, when eaten on a daily basis in one to three gram amounts, is not in its protein food value, but instead is in a 'controlled growth factor'—designated as 'CGF' by Japanese biochemists to describe the combination of molecules that provide a large increase in sustaining energy when certain types of algae are eaten by man..."

CGF is not a single substance, but contains a variety of substances such as amino acids, peptides (like glutathione), proteins, vitamins, sugars, and nucleic acid–related substances such as adenosine nucleotide and cytidine nucleotide.

But That's Not All

Chlorella contains more chlorophyll than any other known plant. It has ten times the amount found in alfalfa.

Chlorophyll is an effective detoxifier for the liver and the bloodstream.

Chlorophyll cleanses the bowels.

Iron is more easily absorbed in the presence of chlorophyll.

Chlorophyll affects nutrition, synthesis of vitamins in plants, hormone action, and wound healing. It aids tissue regeneration and ulcers. It stimulates the body's immune system and helps normalize blood sugar. Chlorophyll is also a splendid deodorant.

All this from a one–celled algae—and there are still more benefits!

The cell–wall material has a special effect on the intestines. It improves bowel function, stimulates the growth of helpful bacteria, and helps to remove poisons from the body.

Fiber helps to stimulate the muscular contractions that move food and waste material through the bowels. This prevents and eliminates constipation. It also keeps toxins in the stool from being reabsorbed into the bloodstream.

Chlorella is able to rid the body of pollutants, even poisons, by actually binding with the toxic agents and removing them from the body with the waste material. It does this with heavy metals, and also with pesticides.

Beneficial bacteria fight off infections and help to detoxify potentially dangerous chemicals in our food. They also help to manufacture some vitamins (B–12 in particular). Chlorella influences the growth of those helpful microbes.

How Can This Little Plant Do All These Things?

One of the reasons is its very high content of chlorophyll. Another possibility is that it is a single cell with a nucleus and resembles the body cells.

Until a few years ago, spirulina was more readily assimilated by the body than chlorella because of the tough cell walls. But, the cell walls were important, so the chlorella manufacturing companies found a way to break down the walls without hindering the efficacy. In this way we are able to get to the nucleus, which spirulina lacks. This is where the nucleic acid, the growth factor, is. The growth factor helps healthy tissue to grow.

Availability: Found in health food stores and drugstores.

Dosage: For weight loss, take three tablets three times a day, or according to manufacturer's directions, before eating and keep your food intake limited to vegetables, cereals, salads, and fruits. Over a period of time, increase your intake of chlorella tablets to five tablets before meals. Drink *at least* eight ounces of water.

If you have unfavorable reactions, discontinue taking them for a few days and then start off with only one tablet before meals. If the reaction continues, you may be one of the unfortunate few who are allergic to chlorella and can't use it.

Chlorella also comes in granule form and in powder form. You can take a teaspoonful of the powder and put it in the blender with six ounces of water. Blend at high speed for four minutes. This mixture can be made and used before meals or as a fasting mixture for a one–day trial, where you would eat no solid food for twenty–four hours.

As with any fast, ask your doctor before you begin.

The "Day Before" Appetite Killer

Some people wake up hungry.

They eat enough at breakfast to carry a normal person through lunch and dinner.

What they have to do is treat themselves to the "Appetite Killer" when they go to bed at night.

It uses natural ingredients that can work with the body's own appetite center. Here's the mixture:

Vitamin C 1,000 mg

L–phenylalanine 500 mg

Vitamin B–6 100 mg

Take these on an empty stomach just before bedtime.

NOTE: There are some people who should not be taking L–phenylalanine. If your doctor says you are one of them, try substituting 500 mg of L–tyrosine. The results will be the same.

If you find that either formula cuts your appetite, you might want to use it twice a day. However, no matter what you use, make sure that one meal a day is a balanced meal with some protein, some carbohydrates, and a bit of oil.

Include some raw vegetables to provide natural enzymes and natural fiber.

Eat smart!

Almost every health food store or drug store carries a good brand of vitamins and amino acids. You don't have to pay for the brand name, but neither should you go by price alone. Ask the person behind the counter for a quality product that he trusts and you should end up with a product that will do the job.

Lose Weight "Fast"

Since fasting was mentioned, there should be some guidelines. Any fast other than a fruit– and vegetable–juice fast should not begin without a consultation with your doctor.

Some people claim that a fast that uses juices is not a "real" fast. In actuality, it's a superior form of fasting. Juices can accelerate the body's cleansing capacity by supplying necessary minerals and ions.

It's a good idea to prepare your body first by going on a two–or–three–day diet. For those days you would eat only fruits and vegetables. The vegetables should be raw for the most part. You'll be surprised at how delicious raw broccoli and raw mushrooms are. Eat fruit for one meal and eat vegetables the next. Do not mix fruit and vegetables at the same meal, because they need different enzymes in order to be digested.

On the fourth day, you can begin your juice fast and, depending on how you feel, stay on it from three to six days.

Your hunger pangs will gradually begin to disappear. Drink as much juice as you can, because the more you drink, the more you will experience a cleansing action, and feel less hunger.

Do not mix fruit juices and vegetables juices.

Carrot juice is great. So is celery juice. Try apple juice and watermelon juice.

Once the fast is over you can return to a normal diet—but do so slowly. Eat small amounts of food when you begin to consume solids. Eat slowly and chew the food thoroughly. Begin with raw fruit and raw vegetables then gradually include other foods.

Some people maintain their weight by fasting for one week every month or every other month.

Cellulite

And now to the "end"—Cellulite, often called "hard–to–budge pudge," that foam–rubber–like deposit of fat that means no more short bathing suits.

Although I have not found any method to remove this ugly mess,

Durk Pearson and Sandy Shaw suggest that cellulite sufferers try 1000 IU per day of vitamin E, plus a powerful free–radical–scavenging formula, such as shown below. It takes at least a year, but some people have said it worked.

No guarantees, but they think it's worth a try.

Vitamin A	5,000 to 8,000 IU
Vitamin B–1	30 to 60 mg
Vitamin B–2	50 to 100 mg
Vitamin B–3	50 to 100 mg
Vitamin B–5	100 to 300 mg
Vitamin B–6	50 to 100 mg
Vitamin B–12	200 to 500 mcg
Vitamin C	1,000 to 5,000 mg
Ascorbyl palmitate	100 mg
Vitamin D	400 IU
Vitamin E	400 to 1,000 IU
Biotin	500 mcg to 1,000 mcg
Beta–carotene	15,000 IU
Cysteine	100 to 300 mg
Folic acid	500 mcg
Hesperidin	150 to 250 mg
PABA	250 mg
Rutin	150 mg
GTF chromium	25 to 100 mcg
Copper	3 to 5 mg in chelated form
Iodine	150 mcg
Manganese	2.5 to 5 mg in chelated form
Molybdenum	150 mcg
Selenium	50 to 150 mcg
Zinc	30 to 50 mg in chelated form

This formula does not have to be followed exactly in the quantities indicated, since each person is an individual with individual needs. Try to take the daily amounts in four equal parts, one dose after each meal and one dose at bedtime.

If you find any distress, start with much smaller quantities and add a little more each week. If distress continues, you may be allergic to either the amount or possibly one of the supplements. If so, try a different formula.

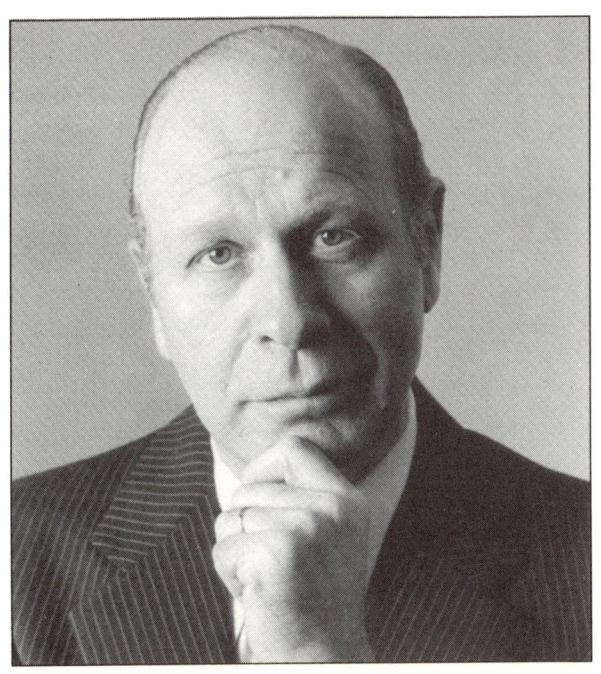

About the Author

William H. Lee, R.Ph., Ph.D is a registered pharmacist, herbalist, and nutritionalist. He is the author of *Concentrated Healing Foods*, Instant Improvement, New York; *New Power to Love*, Instant Improvement, New York; *The Book of Raw Fruit and Vegetable Juices and Drinks*, Keats Publishing, New Cannan, Connecticut. He has written many other books and pamphlets for professionals and for the general public, including *Herbs and Herbal Medicine, Kelp, Dulse and Other Sea Supplements, The Question and Answer Book of Vitamins, The Medicinal Benefits of Mushrooms*, and the *How Do I Know If I Need Vitamins and If I Do—Which One?* handbook.

He is also the author of numerous articles for health food publications, and is the nutrition columnist for *American Druggist*.

Dr. Lee, a native of Canada, has lived most of his life in New York City. He received his pharmaceutical degree from St. John's University and then continued his education in Europe. He and his wife reside in New York's Greenwich Village, where he conducts his consultation service for the direct marketing industry and for a chain of health food stores.

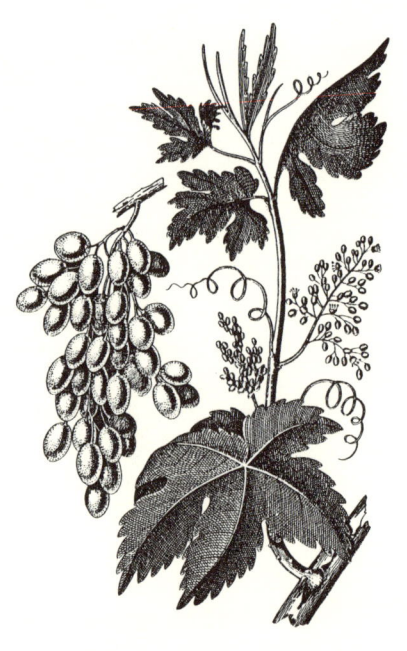

Bibliography

Adams, Ruth, and Frank Murray. *All You Should Know About Health Foods.* Atlanta, GA: Communication Channels, 1983.

Airola, Paavo. *How to Get Well.* Scottsdale, AZ: Health Plus Publishers, 1987.

— *The Miracle of Garlic.* Scottsdale, AZ: Health Plus Publishers, 1987.

— *Worldwide Secrets for Staying Young.* Scottsdale, AZ: Health Plus Publishers, 1982.

Bell, H., and others. *Textbook of Physiology and Biochemistry.* Baltimore, MD: Williams and Wilkins, 1965.

Benowicz, Robert J. *Vitamins and You.* New York: Berkley Publishing Group, 1984.

Burtis, E.C. *Nature's Miracle Medicine.* New York: Arco Publishing, 1971.

Challem, J.J. *Spirulina: What It Is--The Health Benefits It Can Give You.* New Canaan, CT: Keats Publishing Inc., 1981.

Chase, A. *Nutrition for Health.* West Nyack, NY: Parker Publishing Co., 1954.

Cheraskin, E., and W.M. Ringsdorff, Jr. *Psychodietetics.* New York: Bantam Books Inc., 1976.

Colbin, Annemarie. *Food and Healing.* New York: Ballantine/Del Rey/Fawcett Books, 1986.

Colgan, Michael. *Your Personal Vitamin Profile: A Medical Scientist Shows You How to Chart Your Individual Vitamin and Mineral Formula.* New York: William Morrow & Co., 1982.

Cureton, Thomas Kirk. *Physiological Effects of Wheat Germ Oil on Humans in Exercise: Forty-two Physical Training Programs Utilizing 894 Humans.* Springfield, IL: Charles C. Thomas, Publisher, 1972.

Fredericks, Carlton. *Eat Well and Stay Well.* New York: Grosset & Dunlap, 1980.

— *Carlton Fredericks' Program for Living Longer.* New York: Simon & Schuster, Inc., 1983.

— *Psycho-Nutrition.* New York: Grosset & Dunlap, 1972.

Gelenberg, A.J., and others. "Tyrosine for the Treatment of Depression." *American Journal of Psychiatry,* 147 (May 1980): 622-623.

Goldberg, I. "Tyrosine in Depression." *The Lancet.* (August, 1980).

Goodhart, R.S., and M.E. Shils. *Modern Nutrition in Health and Disease.* 6th edition. Philadelphia: Lea & Febiger, 1980.

Hanssen, M. *Spirulina: Nature's Diet Supplement Rediscovered.* Wellingborough, Northants, England: Thorsons Publishers, 1982.

Huttunen, J.K. "Fructose in Medicine. A Review with Particular Reference to Diabetes Mellitus." *Postgraduate Medical Journal,* 45 (1971): 654-659.

Kovisto, V.A. "Fructose as a Dietary Sweetener in Diabetes." *Diabetes Care* 1 (July/August 1978).

Lehninger, A.L. *Biochemistry.* New York: Worth Publishers, 1978.

Lesser, Michael, M.D. *Nutrition and Vitamin Therapy.* New York: Bantam Books Inc., 1981.

McCormick, M. *The Golden Pollen.* Yakima, WA: Yakima Printing Co., 1960.

Mann, J.A. *Secrets of Life Extension.* San Francisco: Harbor Publishing, 1980.

Marks, V.A., and E. Samols. "Intestinal Factors in the Regulation of Insulin Secretion." In *Advances in Metabolic Medicine,* edited by R. Levine and R. Luft, 4:1. New York: Academic Press, 1970.

Mertz, W. "The Essential Trace Elements." *Science* 213: 1332-1338.

Mindell, Earl. *Earl Mindell's New and Revised Vitamin Bible*. New York: Warner Books Inc., 1985.

— *Shaping Up With Vitamins*. New York: Warner Books Inc., 1985.

Offenbacher, E., and others. "Beneficial Effects of Chromium-rich Yeast on Glucose Tolerance and Blood Lipids in Elderly Subjects." *Diabetes* 29 (November 1980): 919-925.

Passwater, Richard A. *Cancer and Its Nutritional Treatment*. New Canaan, CT: Keats Publishing Inc., 1978.

— *Evening Primrose Oil*. New Canaan, CT: Keats Publishing Inc., 1981.

— *GTF Chromium*. New Canaan, CT: Keats Publishing Inc., 1982.

— *Supernutrition*. New York: Pocket Books, 1975.

Pearson, Durk, and Sandy Shaw. "How to Prevent Jet Lag." *Anti-aging News*. (February 1981).

— *Life Extension*. New York: Warner Books Inc., 1983.

Robinson, C.H. *Normal and Therapeutic Nutrition*. New York: Macmillan Publishing Co., 1972.

Rose, W.C. "Amino Acid Requirements of Man." *Nutrition Review* 34 (1967): 307-309.

Scala, James. *Making the Vitamin Connection*. New York: Harper & Row, Publishers, Inc., 1985.

Schroeder, H.A. "The Role of Chromium in Mammalian Nutrition." *American Journal of Clinical Nutrition* 21 (1980): 230-244.

Shaffer, R.E. "Durk Pearson Shares Secrets of Life Extension." *The Journal of the International Academy of Nutritional Consultants* (November/December 1980).

Smith, G.P., and J. Gibbs. "Brain-gut Peptides and the Control of Food Intake." In *Neurosecretion and Brain Peptides: Implications for Brain Function and Neurologic Disease*. New York: Raven Press, 1980.

Switzer, L. *Spirulina: The Whole Food Revolution*. New York: Bantam Books Inc., 1982.

Vaughan, William J. *Low Salt Secrets for Your Diet*. New York: Warner Books Inc., 1984.

Wade, Carlson. *Bee Pollen and Your Health*. New Canaan, CT: Keats Publishing Inc., 1985.

— *Carlson Wade's Amino Acids Book*. New Canaan, CT: Keats Publishing Inc., 1985.

— *Lecithin Book*. New Canaan, CT: Keats Publishing Inc., 1980.

— *Vitamins, Minerals and Other Supplements*. New Canaan, CT: Keats Publishing Inc., 1983.

Williams, Roger J. *Nutrition Against Disease*. White Plains, NY: Pitman/Longman Inc., 1971.

Wurtman, R.J. "Nutrients That Modify Brain Function." *Scientific American* (April 1982): 50-59.

— and J.J. Wurtman. *Nutrition and the Brain*. New York: Raven Press, 1979.

Index

L–glutamine 26–28
L–ornithine 49–50, 119–120
L–phenylalanine 22–25, 42, 55,
   119–120, 131–132, 137–138, 141, 158
L–tyrosine 25–26, 42, 55, 120, 133, 138,
   158
LDL 79
lactic acid 37–38
laxatives 138–139, 154
lecithin 100–104
liver, the 16, 23–34, 41–45, 81–85,
   155–158
lungs, the 16

M

MAO 24
meats 20, 21, 25–26, 45, 73–76, 105–118,
   125–135, 137, 151–159
metabolism 13, 14, 15, 22–34, 35–45,
   47–50, 51–65, 67–72, 73–76, 77–79,
   81–104, 105–118, 119–120, 121–124,
   125–135, 137–143, 151–159
methylcellulose 51–65
milk 20, 21, 25–26, 45, 68–72, 73–76,
   105–118, 137–143, 151–159
minerals 15, 23–34, 35–45, 47–50,
   51–65, 68–72, 75–76, 78–79, 81–85,
   87–104, 155–158
muscles, the 16, 36–38, 41–45, 47–50,
   68–73, 78–79, 87–104, 105–118,
   119–120, 125–135, 137–143, 152–159

N

neurotransmitters 19, 20, 21, 22–23,
   25–34, 88–104, 119–120, 125–135,
   137–143, 151–159
"new brain" 15
nitrogen 20
noradrenaline 22–24, 25–26
nutrient formulas 87–104
nutrients 17, 19, 20, 21, 23–34, 35–45,
   47–50, 51–65, 67–72, 73–76, 81–85,
   87–104, 105–118, 119–120, 125–135,
   137–143, 151–159

O

octacosanol 88–104, 125
oil of evening primrose 70–72, 142–143
"old brain" 15
oxygen 16, 36–38

P

PKU 24
pectin 133–134
phenylalanine 21–24, 55–65
phosphosugar 40–42
pituitary gland, the 39–40, 48–50
prostaglandins 67–72
protein 15, 20, 41–45, 49–50, 78–79,
   82–85, 87–104, 105–118, 125–135,
   137–143, 151–159
pyrodoxine (see: vitamin B–6)

R

rice 20

S

salt substitutes 153–154
seaweed 81–85
selenium 40, 75–76
spirulina 51–65, 88–104
sugars 16, 26–34, 40–42, 54–65, 77–79,
   87–104, 133, 134
supplements 20, 21, 22, 23–34, 35–45,
   47–50, 54–65, 67–72, 73–76, 77–79,
   81–85, 87–104, 105–118, 119–120,
   125–135, 137–143, 152–159

T

thyroid (gland) 13, 81–85, 151–154
thyroxine 23–24
trace elements 15